The Complete Idiot's Refer[ence]

Top Five Exercise Tips

1. Set realistic goals. Aim to look and feel *your* best—not somebody else's best.
2. Pace yourself. It's much better to consistently work out three times per week for 30 minutes each session, than to come on strong with two-hour sessions for seven straight days, only to drop out of sight for the next two months.
3. Vary your workouts. Don't get caught up in the same exercise routine day in and day out!
4. Keep yourself properly hydrated. Drink plenty of water before, during, and after exercising.
5. Make exercise fun and convenient—*not* a hassle. Do what works best for you and your schedule, whether it means joining a gym, buying home equipment, or simply walking home from work. If planned exercise is just not your thing, go ahead and break it up into three 10-minute bouts throughout the day—you'll still get the health benefits!

Top Five Nutrition Tips

1. Eat plenty of whole grain products. Breads, cereal, pasta, and rice provide B-vitamins and lots of complex carbohydrates.
2. Fill up on fresh fruit and veggies. They are *loaded* with nutrients and are naturally low in fat and calories.
3. Make it a habit to choose low-fat dairy. Low-fat milk, yogurts, and cheese supply protein and *calcium*—a key ingredient for building and maintaining strong, healthy bones.
4. Stick with the lean sources of protein. Some sources include chicken breast, turkey breast, lean red meats, seafood and fish, egg whites, tofu, beans, and legumes.
5. Take it easy on the fat and sugar. Limit your intake of fried foods, butter, margarine, cream, salad dressings, oils, sugars, soft drinks, rich desserts, candies, cakes, cookies, and so on.

Calories in Commonly Eaten Foods

Food	Calories
Bread, (1 slice)	67
Crackers, (5)	60
Bagel, (1 medium)	234
Apple, (1 medium)	80
Strawberries, (1 cup)	45
Banana, (1 medium)	105
Orange juice, (1 cup)	110
Broccoli,(cooked, 1/2 cup)	25
Carrot, (1 whole)	31
Corn, (1/2 cup)	67
1% low-fat milk, (1 cup)	102
Low-fat fruit yogurt, (1 cup)	230
Non-fat fruit yogurt, (1 cup)	140
Steak, lean, (5 ounces)	293
Chicken breast, (5 ounces)	233
Hot dog, (with bun)	294
Hamburger, (with bun)	393
Cheeseburger, (with bun)	520
Jelly beans, (30)	198
Chocolate chip cookies, (3)	158
Soda, (12 ounces)	151

Calories Burned During Popular Exercises

The following list represents the *approximate* calories spent per hour by a 100-pound and 150-pound person doing a particular activity. The actual number of calories you burn will vary in proportion to your body weight and the intensity of your workout.

	100 lb.	150 lb.
Bicycling, 6 mph	160	240
Bicycling, 12 mph	270	410
Jogging, 5 1/2 mph	440	660
Jogging, 7 mph	610	920
Jumping rope	500	750
Running, 10 mph	850	1,280
Running in place	430	650
Swimming, 25 yds./min.	185	275
Swimming, 50 yds./min.	325	500
Tennis, singles	265	400
Walking, 2 mph	160	240
Walking, 3 mph	210	320
Walking, 4 1/2 mph	295	440

Source; American Heart Association

tear here

alpha
books

Nutrition/Fitness Health Directory

The American Dietetic Association
National Center for Nutrition and Dietetics (NCND)
216 West Jackson Blvd.
Chicago, IL 60606
Consumer Nutrition Hotline:(800) 366-1655

Food Research & Action Center (FRAC)
1875 Connecticut Ave. NW
Suite 540
Washington, DC 20009
(202) 986-2200

Public Voice for Food and Health Policy
1101 14th Street NW
Suite 710
Washington, DC 20005
(202) 371-1840

American Heart Association
National Center
7272 Greenville Ave.
Dallas, TX 75231-4596
(800) AHA-USA1 (800) 242-8721

American Cancer Society
1599 Clifton Road. NE
Atlanta, GA 30329
(800) 227-2345

American Institute for Cancer Research
1759 R Street NW
Washington, DC 20009
(800) 843-8114

American Health Foundation
1 Dana Road
Valhalla, NY 10595
(914) 789-7122

The Food Allergy Network
10400 Eaton Place
Suite 107
Fairfax, VA 22030
(800) 929-4040

Arthritis Foundation Information Line
1314 Spring Street NW
Atlanta, GA 30309
(800) 283-7800

American Diabetes Association
1660 Duke Street
Alexandria, VA 22314
(800) DIABETES (800) 342-2383

Celiac Disease Foundation
13251 Ventura Blvd.
Suite 1
Studio City, CA 91604
(818) 990-2354

National Association of Anorexia Nervosa & Associated
Disorders (ANAD)
P.O. Box 7
Highland Park, IL 60035
(847) 831-3438

American Anorexia/Bulimia Association
293 Central Park West, Suite #1R
New York, NY 10024
(212) 501-8351

National Eating Disorders Organization
Laureate Eating Disorder Unit
6655 South Yale Avenue
Tulsa, OK 74136
(918) 481-4044

Aerobics and Fitness Association of America (AFAA)
15250 Ventura Blvd.
Suite 200
Sherman Oaks, CA 91403
(800) 446-2322

The International Association of Fitness
Professionals(IDEA)
6190 Cornerstone Ct. East
Suite 204
San Diego, CA 92121
(800) 999-IDEA

In addition, the following two organizations publish a
monthly newsletter reporting current nutrition information:

Center for Science in the Public Interest
1875 Connecticut Ave. NW
Suite 300
Washington, DC 20009
Nutrition Action Health Letter
(800) 237-4874

Tufts University Diet and Nutrition Letter
6 Beacon Street
Suite 1110
Boston, MA 02108
(800) 274-7581

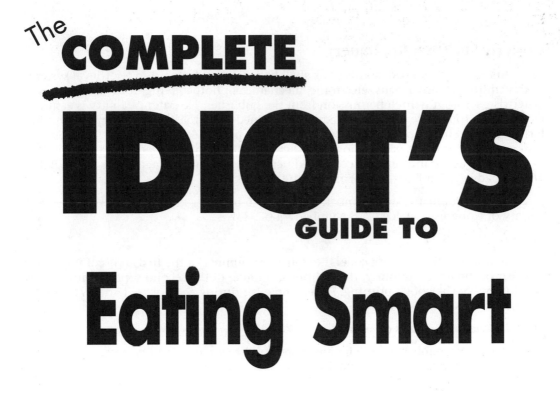

The COMPLETE IDIOT'S GUIDE TO Eating Smart

by Joy Bauer

alpha
books

A Division of Macmillan General Reference
A Simon & Schuster Macmillan Company
1633 Broadway, 7th Floor, New York NY 10019

Publisher
Theresa Murtha

Editor
Nancy Mikhail

Production/Copy Editor
Brian Robinson

Cover Designer
Michael Freeland

Illustrator
Judd Winick

Designer
Glenn Larsen

Indexer
Becky Hornyak

Production Team
Angela Calvert
Tricia Flodder
Laure Robinson
Megan Wade

Contents at a Glance

Contents

Foreword

Whether you are at a restaurant, a party, an office building, the movies, a wedding, or a funeral; whether you are in the East, West, South, or North, everyone talks about *IT*, everyone has to do *IT*, we usually feel good doing *IT*, and if we overdo *IT*, we see the consequences. Poor choices of *IT* can lead to some serious medical conditions. Of course, *IT* is EATING. Just about everyone knows that eating healthy is important for overall health and well-being. We can prevent or reduce the risk of certain conditions such as obesity, hypertension, and osteoporosis by making smart food choices early in life and continuing through adulthood. Sometimes, however, the information about food and nutrition gets confusing, and you hear many different opinions. What exactly are RDA, FDA, CHO, PRO, DV., cc's., and kcal?

Who can possibly make this nutrition jargon palatable (bad pun) for the public? Not many people can, but Joy Bauer certainly does in her book, *The Complete Idiot's Guide to Eating Smart.* Joy's charm, knowledge, and wit shine through in all of her chapters. This book focuses on eating healthy for every age, and also includes useful information about behavior, emotions, and individual differences. You will laugh out loud at some of the questions that you wondered about, but never received an answer to, such as:

> ➤ Are all fats created equal?

> ➤ What do all those cholesterol numbers mean?

> ➤ Must you have milk during pregnancy?

> ➤ Do you need extra protein for weight training?

> ➤ Is it really possible not to gain the "freshman fifteen?"

> ➤ Chinese food is really healthy, right?

> ➤ Am I burning fat after 30 minutes of walking on a treadmill?

> ➤ I don't eat that much, but why can't I lose weight?

> ➤ Is tofu really that good for you or is it just a trend?

> ➤ After reading *The Complete Idiot's Guide to Eating Smart*, you will be able to answer these questions and understand how the answers apply to you.

Joy Bauer brings to you the essence of her years of knowledge from her work at Mount Sinai Medical Center, her teaching at New York University, and her lecturing throughout New York City. Joy is recognized not only as a nutritionist with an extensive background in couseling, but a person with great empathy and compassion. She makes every person she "touches" feel wonderful about themselves. Joy passes on the message of healthy eating in her book with the same flair. You will learn, laugh, and most importantly, understand how healthy eating can be incorporated into your life, so you feel as good as you possibly can.

Elyse Sosin, R.D.

Elyse has earned a Master of Arts and a Bachelor of Science degree in nutrition. She is the nutritionist at the Women's Health Program at Mount Sinai Medical Center. She currently co-directs a Cardiovascular Risk Reduction program for teens, and provides nutritional guidance for teenagers at the Adolescent Health Center at Mount Sinai Medical Center. Elyse is the nutrition counselor for the CHOICE program at the Adolescent Heatlth Center, which treats teens with eating disorders. High risk pregnancy and Gestational Diabetes counseling round out her care for women.

Elyse is a lecturer for the American Heart Association and Mount Sinai's Wellness Program. Her topics often include weight reduction, cardiovascular risk reduction for teens, healthy eating, and eating disorders.

Elyse has a private practice in Manhattan.

Introduction

Sometimes it seems that you have to be a genius to sort through the enormous amount of nutrition information bombarding us on a daily basis. Constantly fed with conflicting stories from the government, media, and, of course, loving friends and relatives, how is anyone supposed to make sense of what's what in the world of healthful eating? Over the course of my career I've seen and heard it all: the vitamin pill poppers, the fad diet groupies, the fat-phobic generation, the protein shakers, and the people that live life according to the "seafood diet"—they *see food* and they eat it!

So what is good eating anyway? Good eating requires all foods in moderation, balance, and variety. It's about making a life-long commitment to nourishing your body with quality fuel. It requires understanding the fundamentals of carbohydrates, protein, and fat. Furthermore, you need to understand that you must eat the right proportions to look and feel your best.

In this book, you will finally find a comprehensive guide to eating smart and becoming fit that is not only up-to-date, but trustworthy, and most importantly, reader-friendly! It was written with both my personal and professional experiences in mind, for people who want to slim down, bulk up, or just plain look and feel great.

How to Use this Book

To make the reading easier for you, I've divided these pages into seven areas of interest.

Part 1, Understanding Nutrition Today: This section clears up the confusion on the fundamentals of food. It dissects the food guide pyramid and offers simple strategies to incorporate the five food groups into your diet. You'll also get the inside scoop on simple to complex carbohydrates, the power of protein, and the relationship between excessive fat intake and heart disease. In addition, you'll examine the facts on fiber and salt, plus become well-versed on the vital vitamins and minerals that your body requires.

Part 2, Making Savvy Food Choices: Here, you'll learn that dining healthy does not mean giving up the pleasure of eating. In this section you'll get the insight to become Sherlock Holmes in your grocery store, able to decode the nutrition information on product labels and make better informed food purchases. We'll take a trial run through the supermarket and load your cart with smart food items to stock in your kitchen. You'll also be supplied with lots of easy-to-make and creative recipes, and learn to master the art of low-fat cooking. Further, I'll provide the best bets in nearly every ethnic cuisine so you'll be ready to tackle any type of restaurant.

Part 3, Learning the ABCs of Exercise: This part provides you with the tools and inspiration to get moving and keep moving. That's right, a crash course on becoming physically fit. You'll hear the lowdown on strengthening your heart and lungs through aerobic exercise and tips to buff your soon-to-be bodacious physique through appropriate weight training and conditioning. You'll learn the importance of properly warming up, cooling down, and stretching your body, *plus* get the education needed to enter a gym with confidence. I'll also take a comprehensive look at sports nutrition and provide the skills you'll need to fuel your body for both casual exercise and competitive sport.

Part 4, Nutrition Sidelines: This area supplies a complete guide to vegetarianism for the vegans, lactos, ovolactos, and pseudo-vegetarians out there. This section will also zoom in on the common culprits that trigger food allergies, food intolerances, and other food-related hypersensitivities.

Part 5, Healthy Kids: From the Cradle to College Graduation: In these chapters you'll find surefire tips to help get your kids eating healthy foods. This section includes lower-fat afterschool snack ideas, strategic ways to disguise vegetables, and tips to encourage more physical activity. I'll also address the college crowd and map out best bites in the campus dining hall, the real-deal on vending machines, late night munchies, alcohol and partying, and of course, how to avoid those notorious "freshman fifteen" pounds of weight that seem to creep up on a lot of college students.

Part 6, Pregnancy: Nutrition and Fitness for Two: I'll provide essential information that will help manage you and your growing baby's health. I'll discuss the importance of sound nutrition and offer specific food guidelines for a healthy pregnancy. You'll learn how much weight you should gain, the right foods to eat, and which foods to avoid. This section will also fill you in on the dos and don'ts of appropriate exercise during pregnancy.

Part 7, Weight Management 101: This section provides you with a sensible plan of attack. Whether you want to lose weight, gain weight, or most importantly, stop obsessing, this final section covers it all. I'll provide weight loss programs to help knock off (and keep off) those extra unwanted pounds, along with calorie-cramming strategies to help you skinny folks beef up your bods. I'll also take a look at life-threatening eating disorders, and where to find help when food and exercise go beyond health and get way out of control.

Extras

To help you get the most out of this book, I've sprinkled it with the following helpful information boxes:

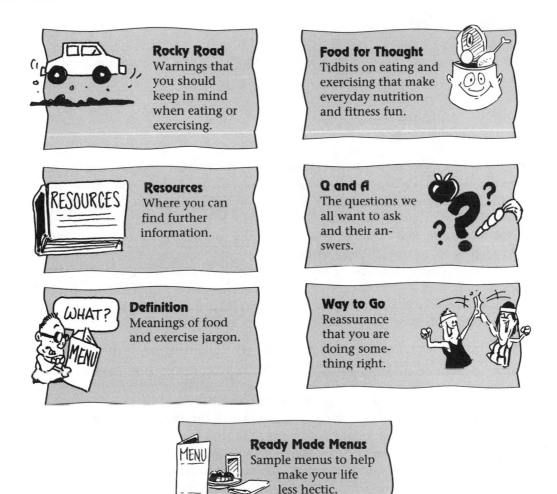

Rocky Road
Warnings that you should keep in mind when eating or exercising.

Food for Thought
Tidbits on eating and exercising that make everyday nutrition and fitness fun.

Resources
Where you can find further information.

Q and A
The questions we all want to ask and their answers.

Definition
Meanings of food and exercise jargon.

Way to Go
Reassurance that you are doing something right.

Ready Made Menus
Sample menus to help make your life less hectic.

Dedication

This book is dedicated to my husband Ian, and daughter Jesse, who are always there to make me smile.

Acknowledgments

Many thanks to my wonderful literary agent Mitch Douglas, who gave me the chance to create this book. Also, special thanks go to the following: Nancy Mikhail, my talented and enthusiastic editor; Brian Robinson, my creative production editor; Michael Simon, the man who always puts me in touch with the right people; Meredith Gunsberg for her invaluable input; and Geralyn Coopersmith and Evan Spinks, two outstanding fitness consultants who shared their expertise and sense of humor. In addition, I'm grateful to many others who contributed to portions of this book, including Elyse Sosin, M.A. R.D., Grace Leder, Meg Fein, Dany Levy, Candy Gulko, Jane Stern, Vanessa Grigoriadis, Dr. Catharine Fedeli, Dr. Susan Wagner, Betsy Keller, M.S. R.D., Lisa Delaney, M.S. R.D., and Heidi Skolnik, M.S.

On a personal note, I would like to extend a sincere thanks to my loving family and friends: my incredible parents Ellen and Artie Schloss, who have always taught me that *anything* and *everything* is possible; my grandma Martha for promising she'd stick around to see my book published; "The gang," Debra, Steve, Glenn, Pam, Dan, Nancy, Jon, Harley, Lisa, and Jason (Dan and Steve, thanks for all the expert advice and cheap services); Lisa Alexander for showering my daughter with love and care; my super in-laws, Carol and Vic, along with grandma Mary and grandpa Nat, for their support and encouragement. Most of all, I want to thank my wonderful husband Ian, and beautiful daughter Jesse, for constantly nourishing me with love, and making my life everything I could ever hope for.

Part 1
Understanding Nutrition Today

After reading and listening to conflicting food advice from friends, relatives, and mailmen (yes, even my mailman, Marty, once tried to tell me to drink carrot juice for thicker hair), it's no wonder people are more confused than ever about what they should be eating.

This first part of the book proves that eating healthy does need not be complicated or restrictive. In fact, it is quite the contrary. This section unravels the colorful food guide pyramid, and provides the inside scoop on carbohydrates, protein, fat, fiber, and salt. After grasping these fundamentals of food, you'll be ready to read further into the book and learn the specifics about everything you never understood or realized. Okay, let's get the ball rolling!

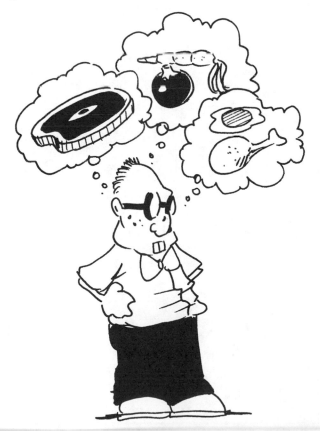

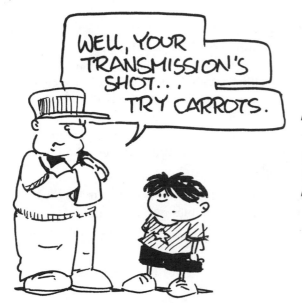

Chapter 1

Time for a Nutrition Tune-Up!

In This Chapter

➤ Unraveling the Food Guide Pyramid

➤ Balancing out your food groups

➤ Where do calories fit in?

➤ The keys to successful eating

➤ Scheduling time to fuel your body

After palming through hundreds of complicated nutrition articles and magazine ads, tuning in to piecemeal food advice from friends and relatives, and listening warily to endless infomercials promising an instantly bodacious bod (just add water), you're probably more confused than ever about what the heck you should be eating. *So, what exactly should you be eating?*

Believe it or not, healthy eating does not involve driving miles out of your way in search of organic produce in some obscure health food store. It also doesn't mean eating bean sprouts sprinkled with wheat germ for dinner (umm, umm). Whew, that's a relief, huh? In fact, according to nutrition experts, healthy eating is more basic than you think.

Solving the Pyramid Puzzle

In 1992, the United States Department of Agriculture (USDA) created the *Food Guide Pyramid*, which is an updated version of the familiar basic four food groups that have been drilled into your head since the first grade. I'm sure you've seen this colorful Egyptian triangle on the packages of products in the grocery store and on the back of your favorite cereal box. This fun, visual approach to nutrition makes healthy eating a lot less complicated, providing a general outline of what you should eat each day. While individuals vary in their specific requirements, the food guide pyramid provides solid information on do's and don'ts for the general population.

The Food Guide Pyramid emphasizes eating a variety of foods from the five main food groups. (That's right—the USDA separated fruits and vegetables into two different groups.) It also limits the amount of fats, oils, and sweets in your diet. Here's the cast list:

Group 1: Breads, Cereal, Rice, and Pasta

Group 2: Vegetable

Group 3: Fruit

Group 4: Milk, Yogurt, and Cheese

Group 5: Meat, Poultry, Fish, Dry Beans, Eggs, and Nuts

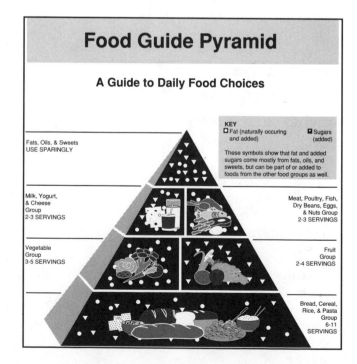

4

Let's take a peek at how this model works:

1. **Breads, Cereal, Rice, and Pasta Group:** Foods that come from grains sit at the bottom of the pyramid, creating a foundation to build a healthy diet on. This foundation provides vitamins and minerals, along with complex carbohydrates (also called carbs or carbos), which serve as an important source of energy. To add some fiber to your diet, eat whole grains whenever possible. USDA guidelines recommend 6–11 servings per day. That may sound like a lot, but serving sizes are deceptively small, so they add up quickly!

   One serving = 1 slice of bread,

   > $1/_2$ English muffin, 1 hamburger roll, small bagel, ounce of ready to eat cereal, one tortilla
   > or
   > $1/_2$ cup cooked cereal, rice, or pasta

2. **Vegetable Group:** Depending on which ones you choose, veggies are loaded with vitamins and minerals, including vitamins A and C, folate, iron, magnesium, and several others. Vegetables are naturally low in calories and fat, plus packed with fiber (bonus!). USDA guidelines recommend 3–5 servings per day.

   One serving = 1 cup of raw leafy vegetables,

   > $1/_2$ cup cooked or chopped, or
   >
   > $3/_4$ cup vegetable juice

3. **Fruit Group:** Fruits and fruit juices are terrific sources of vitamins A and C and potassium. Eat whole fruits often—they are higher in fiber than juice. USDA guidelines recommend 2–4 servings per day.

   One serving = 1 medium whole fruit (apple, banana, orange)

   > $3/_4$ cup of unsweetened fruit juice,
   >
   > $1/_2$ grapefruit,
   >
   > $1/_2$ cup of chopped, canned, or cooked fruit,
   >
   > $1/_4$ cup dried fruit, or wedge of melon

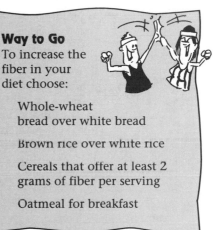

Way to Go
To increase the fiber in your diet choose:

Whole-wheat bread over white bread

Brown rice over white rice

Cereals that offer at least 2 grams of fiber per serving

Oatmeal for breakfast

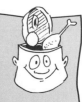

Food for Thought
Look how quickly the grains can add up:

Bet ya didn't know that…

a pasta entree = 4–5 grain servings

a large New York bagel = 3–4 servings

a large hot pretzel = 3 servings

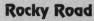

Rocky Road

When buying fruit juice, pay close attention to the wording on the juice containers—they may not be as healthy as they sound. For instance, "Fruit Drinks" and "Fruit Cocktails" generally contain lots of added sugar with small amounts of real fruit juice. Instead of falling for these impostors, examine the label and select fruit beverages that read "100% Fruit Juice."

4. **Milk, Yogurt, and Cheese Group:** The hands-down winners of the calcium contest, these foods also provide protein and other vitamins and minerals. USDA guidelines recommend 2–3 servings per day—two for most people and three for teenagers, young adults under 24, and women who are pregnant or breast-feeding.

One serving = 1 cup of milk or yogurt, 1 $1/_2$–2 ounces of cheese, or 1 cup cottage cheese

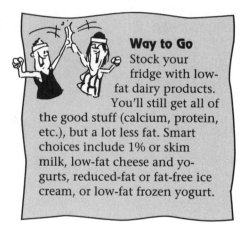

Way to Go
Stock your fridge with low-fat dairy products. You'll still get all of the good stuff (calcium, protein, etc.), but a lot less fat. Smart choices include 1% or skim milk, low-fat cheese and yogurts, reduced-fat or fat-free ice cream, or low-fat frozen yogurt.

5. **Meat, Poultry, Fish, Dry Beans, Eggs, and Nuts Group:** Along with supplying substantial amounts of protein, this group contains B-vitamins, iron, and zinc. USDA guidelines recommend 2–3 servings per day, the equivalent of 5–7 ounces.

One serving = 2–3 ounces of cooked lean meat, or 2–3 ounces of cooked fish or skinless poultry, or Count $1/_2$ cup cooked beans, or 1 egg, or 2 tablespoons peanut butter, or $1/_2$ cup of nuts as 1 ounce lean meat.

Food for Thought
Although eggs are a good source of protein, the yolks contain high amounts of cholesterol. Limit your consumption of egg yolks to 3–4 servings per week. When you do eat eggs, get into the habit of using the egg substitutes (no cholesterol) or mix one whole egg with two or three whites.

Fats, Oils, and Sweets: The tip of the pyramid is reserved for these "nutrient-less" foods. These spreads, oils, and sugary treats, known as "empty calories," literally offer zilch in the form of nutrition. Every shrewd dieter can tolerate a bit of these foods, but many of us eat far too much fat and sugar, and forget about the important groups that make up 99% of the pyramid's foundation. USDA guidelines recommend limiting your intake of salad dressings and oils, cream, butter, margarine, sugars, soft drinks, candies, and rich desserts.

Where Do Calories Fit In?

Practically everyone over the age of 10 has heard the word "calorie"—but few actually understand how calories work in regard to their diet. For some reason, the word calorie gets a very bad rap, when in fact, a calorie is simply the measurement of food as energy. The more calories you eat, the more energy you supply your body with.

All of the foods we eat contain calories, some more than others. The ideal situation involves *taking in the amount of food energy—calories—that your body needs. No more, no less.* Although this is easier said than done, this tightrope walk will help maintain a normal body weight. Unfortunately, it is quite easy to eat more calories than your body actually needs or burns, resulting in weight gain. On the other hand, taking in fewer calories than your body needs can result in weight loss.

How Many Calories Are Right for You?

So how can you find the perfect balance between calories in and calories out? Not by nit-picking over calorie counting, that's for sure! You *should* pay attention to what and how much you eat, but not to the point that you carry a calculator in your bag, ready to whip it out after each bite of food. So many things in life drive us bonkers, we certainly don't need another thing to obsess over.

To get a *rough* idea of how many calories you should be taking in, look at the following chart. This chart only offers three general caloric ranges, so keep in mind that your personal daily requirements may fall somewhere between two that are listed. Remember, everyone is different. Caloric intake will vary depending upon your age, sex, size, and level of activity. After you have selected the caloric amount that seems right for you, simply experiment with the various number of servings in each group (listed underneath your caloric level) until you find what feels most comfortable. Almost everyone should have

Definition

Calorie: The amount of energy food provides. The number of calories a food provides is determined by burning it in a device called a calorimeter and measuring the amount of heat produced. One calorie is equal to the amount of energy needed to raise the temperature of one liter of water one degree Celsius. Carbohydrates and protein contain 4 calories per gram, fat contains 9 calories per gram, and alcohol has 7 calories per gram.

Food for Thought

All calories are not created equal! Although the following foods contain the same amount of calories, notice the difference in nutrition

PACKAGE OF LICORICE ~230 calories; 0 milligrams calcium; 0 protein; 0 IU vitamin D

8–OUNCE FRUIT YOGURT ~230 calories; 350 milligrams calcium; 8 grams protein; 100 IU vitamin D

** Opt for foods rich in nutrients

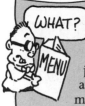

Definitions

Sedentary folks generally have desk jobs, watch lots of TV, and tend to sit around most of the time.

Active folks are constantly on the go. They do lots of walking, taking the stairs, playing sports, and/or regularly working out.

at least the lowest number of servings in the pyramids ranges. You may even want to keep a food log for a week or so—this way you can keep track of the groups you need to increase, and those you may be overloading on.

Leave meticulous measuring and weighing to the folks at Weight Watchers. Remember that serving sizes are approximations, so an eyeball-guess is fine. If you have no idea what a serving size looks like, you may want to measure it out once or twice for a future comparison. For example, measure out a serving of cooked pasta ($^1/_2$ cup) so that you are able to guesstimate that a restaurant entree is probably about 4–5 servings.

Chart 1.1 General Calorie Requirements

1,600 calories	Number of calories needed for many sedentary women and some older adults.
2,200 calories	Number of calories needed for most children, teenage girls, active women, and many sedentary men. Women who are pregnant and breast-feeding may need somewhat more.
2,800 calories	Number of calories needed for teenage boys, many active men, and some very active women.

*Source, USDA 1992

Now that you have an idea of how many calories you should be taking in daily, look at the chart below to determine how many servings of each group will be right for you.

	1,600 calories	2,200 calories	2,800 calories
BREAD GROUP SERVINGS	6	9	11
VEGETABLE GROUP SERVINGS	3	4	5
FRUIT GROUP SERVINGS	2	3	4
MILK GROUP SERVINGS	2–3*	2–3*	2–3*
MEAT GROUP SERVINGS	2	2–3	3

Women who are breast-feeding or pregnant, teenagers and young adults up to age 24, need at least 3 dairy servings daily.

Here are some handy sample menus for each caloric level.

	1,600 Calories	2,200 Calories	2,800 Calories
Breakfast	1 Bowl cereal 1 Cup low-fat milk 1 Slice toast with jam 1 Banana	3 Pancakes 1 Cup berries and some maple syrup 1 Cup low-fat milk	Bowl of cereal with raisins and low-fat milk Large bagel with a smear of cream cheese Glass of orange juice
Lunch	Turkey breast (approx. 2–3 ounces) 2 Slices Swiss cheese 2 Slices whole wheat bread Lettuce and tomato Carrot sticks	Turkey burger on a roll (about 3 ounces) Green salad with vinaigrette	Large salad with 1 cup lentils, small amount of oil and vinegar 1 Slice of broccoli and cheese pizza 1 Apple
Snack	1 Apple	Medium frozen yogurt Banana	2 Fig bars Strawberry yogurt milkshake
Dinner	Salad with vinaigrette Grilled fish (approx. 3 ounces) Rice (approx. 1 cup) Broccoli with parmesan cheese	Sliced tomato and mozzarella (try for low-fat) Linguini (approx. 2 cups)—with shrimp (approx. 3 ounces)—and lots of vegetables in marinara sauce Wedge of melon	1 Dinner roll Lightly stir-fried chicken (approx. 5 ounces)—with lots of vegetables (approx 2 cups) Brown rice (approx. 2 cups) 1 Orange

Adding more tip of the pyramid foods (oil, margarine, dressings, and so on) will increase your daily calories.

The Keys to Successful Eating: Variety, Moderation, and Balance

Now that we've covered the daily food requirements, it's time to get personal and find out what kind of an eater you are. Are you one of those people who orders the exact *same* thing, in the *same* restaurant, day after day? Have you packed the same lunch to bring to work for the last 15 years? Or do you skip eating lunch altogether? Do you define the five food groups as McDonald's, Burger King, Pizza Hut, KFC, and Dunkin Donuts? If you answered "yes" to any of these questions, pay close attention to the next few paragraphs.

Eating a Variety of Healthy Foods

First, understand why variety is important. Varying your food provides a much greater range of nutrients. Eating the same foods day after day, supplies your body with the same exact vitamins and minerals over and over again. While you may be consuming the recommended daily allowance of many beneficial vitamins and minerals, *you miss out on a lot of good stuff that your body needs*. Choose the recommended number of servings from each food group every day.

Furthermore, variety can make your meals much more interesting! Forget about those hum-drum standards. Instead, dare to be adventurous!

➤ Try new cookbooks. Throw things together that you would never have dreamed of eating.

➤ Give your palate a worldly kick. Try a different ethnic restaurant or recipe each week.

➤ Gather a list of 20 different fruits, veggies and grains, and make it your project to try something new each day. Pick one day a week to create a meal that you have never had before. Your tastebuds won't believe what they have been missing!

All Foods in Moderation

We need to place greater emphasis on healthy foods and downplay the not-so-healthy stuff. However, there is a place in *every* food plan for *all* kinds of foods (and let's face it—man cannot live on healthfood alone!). Too many of us label high-fat, high-sugar foods as the enemy, and as a result, feel guilty when we allow ourselves to indulge. Remember, the tip on the pyramid indicates that you should *limit* fat and sugar—not *avoid* it completely.

Take care of your mind as well as your body, if you are absolutely crazy for chocolate cake then you should certainly have the pleasure of eating it once in a while! Obviously, that's not to say that you should eat high fat foods all the time, but there is room for everything *in moderation*. (People who have specific medical conditions such as heart disease, diabetes, food allergies, gastro-intestinal ailments, etc., may have to completely avoid certain foods altogether. Check with your doctor for more information.)

Eating in moderation *also* means controlling the *size* of your portions. Once you have determined the number of servings that you should be eating from each food group, spread them throughout your daily meals. Proper planning will ensure that you are eating balanced meals in moderation, and meeting your daily requirements.

Balancing Out Your Meals with Various Food Groups

Many people eat excessive amounts of food from one group, and completely forget about other groups that offer important vitamins and nutrients. For instance, have you ever watched someone else (*not you, of course*), reach for a couple of rolls from the bread basket, and then polish off a huge plate of pasta? The meal probably tasted delicious, but that's a lot of grain without much of anything else! What happened to the fruits, vegetables, protein, and dairy?

Once in a while, a meal like that is perfectly fine, but as a general rule, incorporate different food groups onto your plate at each meal. For example, choose a house salad, pasta with chicken and broccoli in marinara sauce, and some parmesan cheese. This balanced meal offers a significant amount of nutrition. All you need to do is strategize before throwing something on your plate, and aim for at least two or three food groups with each meal.

Scheduling Time for Breakfast, Lunch, and Dinner

What kind of an eating schedule are you on? Do you make time in your day for breakfast, lunch, and dinner; or do you run on empty until dinner, only to pigout from starvation? Everyone has their own eating regimen, some of which are better than others. However, you should be fueling your bodies *throughout* the day, when you need the energy.

Breakfast with a Bang

You've heard it a million times: BREAKFAST IS IMPORTANT! Think of your body as a car—it needs fuel to run properly. When you wake up from a good night's sleep, your

> **Way to Go**
> "CRASH NUTRITION"
>
> Eat a variety of foods.
>
> Balance the foods you eat with physical activity to maintain or improve your weight.
>
> Choose a diet low in fat, saturated fat, and cholesterol.
>
> Choose a diet with plenty of grain products, vegetables, and fruits.
>
> Choose a diet moderate in sugars, salt, and sodium.
>
> If you drink alcoholic beverages, do so in moderation.
>
> *Developed by The U.S. Departments of Agriculture and Health and Human Services, 1995

body has been in a fasting state for about eight hours (if you're are lucky). "Break-Fast" in the morning helps kick your system into gear by supplying energy in the form of food to your body. Without any food you feel tired and sluggish.

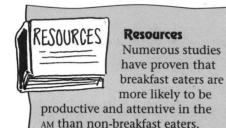

Resources
Numerous studies have proven that breakfast eaters are more likely to be productive and attentive in the AM than non-breakfast eaters.

Incidentally, breakfast also helps you control your weight! Eating a smart breakfast can help regulate your appetite throughout the rest of the day, so you eat in moderation during lunch and dinner. Have you ever skipped breakfast to "save calories," only to find yourself so hungry by lunch that you overeat? So much for that diet! Start your day off smart, schedule time for breakfast.

Fueling Your Body the Rest of the Day

Remember, breakfast alone just won't cut it! Your body needs to be constantly energized throughout the day to help keep you going. You don't necessarily have to eat the standard three square meals. In fact, some prefer six mini-meals (or, constant snacking) each day. Do whatever works best for your schedule and eating style, but be sure that your daily food totals resemble the guidelines of the food guide pyramid.

The Least You Need to Know

➤ Make sure to eat a variety of foods from the five food groups.

➤ Don't get caught up with counting calories—it can drive you crazy! Simply focus on eating foods from all the food groups in moderation.

➤ Get out of your food rut and be adventurous! Try new and exciting foods, recipes, and restaurants.

➤ Although the food pyramid allows for "some" fat and sugar intake, don't overdo it and consume grandiose amounts.

➤ Schedule time to fuel your body *throughout* the day. Food can help keep you alert, energetic, and focused.

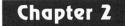

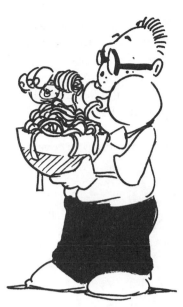

Chapter 2

A Close-Up on Carbohydrates

In This Chapter

➤ What exactly is a carbohydrate?

➤ Simple carbs vs. complex carbs

➤ How many carbohydrates should you eat?

➤ Do starchy carbs make you fat?

➤ To artificially sweeten or not

All of the foods you eat are comprised of three macro-nutrients known as carbohydrate, protein, and fat. Some foods consist primarily of only one macro-nutrient (i.e., bread is mainly carbohydrate, turkey meat is protein, and butter is fat), while other foods contain combinations of all three (for example, pizza, sandwiches, and burritos).

Your body needs all three of these macro-nutrients to properly function, but *not* in equal amounts! Most leading health professionals recommend that we eat a daily diet made up of *55–60 percent carbohydrate, 10–15 percent protein, and less than 30 percent total fat (see figure on following page)*. What's more, by following the general guidelines outlined in the food guide pyramid, you'll automatically be meeting these proportions.

Fifty-five to sixty percent carbohydrates—that's more than half our food coming from a single macro-nutrient. And thanks to growing consumer education about nutrition, many people now recognize the benefits of a carbohydrate-rich diet. Not too long ago, our society placed far too much emphasis on eating excessive protein (steaks, chicken, pork, and so on.). Fortunately, the tide has since turned and we are now paying due attention to our carbohydrate-rich side dishes such as rice, pasta, and vegetables. Remember, carbohydrates provide us with important nutrients and they are an excellent source of energy—specifically for those of us with active lifestyles. This following chapter covers the "real deal" on carbos, from simple to complex!

Breakdown of a Healthy Diet.

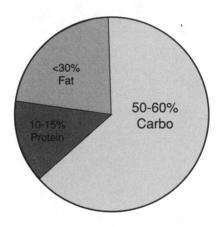

What Exactly Is a Carbohydrate?

Technically speaking, a carbohydrate is a compound made up of carbon, hydrogen, and oxygen—now relax, the technical portion is over. The most basic carbohydrates are called simple sugars, and include honey, jams, jellies, syrup, table sugar, candies, soft drinks, fruits, and fruit juices. As you can see (following figure), they are relatively small compounds. When several of these simple sugars are linked together, they form much more complicated molecules known as complex carbohydrates.

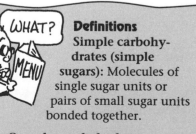

Definitions
Simple carbohydrates (simple sugars): Molecules of single sugar units or pairs of small sugar units bonded together.

Complex carbohydrates (complex sugars): Compounds comprised of long strands of many simple sugars linked together.

Complex carbohydrates that come from plants are called *starch*, and are found in quality foods such as grains, vegetables, breads, seeds, legumes, and beans. So whether it's a handful of jelly beans or freshly sliced whole-grain bread, it's all carbohydrates!

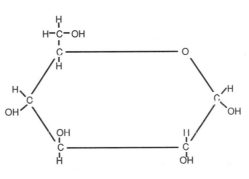

Definition

Legume: Vegetables borne in pods of the bean and pea family that are especially rich in complex carbohydrates, protein, and fiber. They supply iron, zinc, magnesium, phosphorous, potassium, and several B-vitamins, including folic acid. Because foods that fall into this category provide ample amounts of both complex carbs and protein, they can fit in either the meat and beans group *or* the vegetable group. Legumes you may know by more common names include black beans, pinto beans, kidney beans, lima beans, navy beans, soybeans (tofu), black-eyed peas, chickpeas (garbonzos), split peas, lentils, nuts*, and seeds.*

*These are also higher in fat.

A Complex Sugar.

Sweet Satisfaction—The Lowdown on Simple Sugars

So your favorite sugary sweets are classified as carbohydrates—and you're supposed to eat lots of carbohydrates—*so it's okay to load up on gummy bears and licorice, right?* NOT A CHANCE. Here's why.

The *quality* of your carbos matters tremendously! Simple sugars such as candy, sodas, and sugary sweeteners found in cakes and cookies offer little in the form of nutrition except that they provide your body with energy and calories. These foods are literally "empty calories." In moderation, simple sugars are perfectly fine (and I admit, yummy), but people who consistently load up on the sugary sweet stuff often find themselves too full for, or uninterested in, the healthy foods their bodies require. The end result is too much sugar and not enough nutrition.

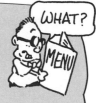

Definition
Empty Calories: Calories with no nutritional value.

Incidentally, sugar can also promote rotting of your teeth. Most of us have heard time and time again from our dentists (and mothers) that excessive sugar can cause cavities. You may roll your eyes, but it's just another argument to limit your sugar intake.

Where Do Fruits and Fruit Juices Fit in?

There are some exceptions to the "no sugar" rule. For example, fruits and fruit juices contain fructose (a natural occurring simple sugar), and in fact both provide several vitamins and minerals. Eating fresh fruit or drinking 100% fruit juice is far from pumping "empty calories" into your system. When possible, try to choose whole fruit over fruit juice since you tend to get the same nutrients, as well as more complex carbohydrates and fiber from the skin and membranes. You'll read more about this in the next chapter.

As you can see by this information, the juice and cola both contain simple sugars, but the juice provides a whole lot more in the way of nutrition.

8 ounces of orange juice supplies	8 ounces of cola supplies
110 calories	100 calories
26 grams carbohydrate	26 grams carbohydrate
25 grams sugar	26 grams sugar
120% daily vitamin C	0% daily vitamin C
12% daily potassium	0% daily potassium
20% daily folic acid	0% daily folic acid

All About Complex Carbohydrates

Now that you know what you *shouldn't* load up on, let's take a look at the foods you *should* eat. You should now be clued in as to which foods are rich in complex carbohydrates (pasta, rice, grains, breads, cereal, legumes, and vegetables). Although they are actually made from hundreds or even thousands of simple sugars linked together, they react quite differently inside your body. After you ingest a complex carbohydrate (or starch), several enzymes break it down into its simplest form, called glucose. Glucose is the simple sugar that your body recognizes and absorbs. All types of carbohydrate (simple and complex) must be broken down and converted into glucose before your body is able to absorb and use it for energy.

If all carbos wind up as glucose, why can't we just eat simple sugars? I've already touched on the first reason: Many simple sugars are nutrition zeroes, whereas complex carbos often provide vitamins, minerals, and even fiber, depending on the food. Check out this comparison, a small baked potato (complex carbo) vs. an 8-ounce glass of cola (simple carbo). Although both provide about 100 calories, that's where the similarity ends. The potato supplies vitamin C, potassium, and fiber, along with several other vitamins and minerals. And the cola—well you probably guessed—*it provides zilch*! As you can see, eating complex carbos certainly does make a difference, even though it all ends up as glucose.

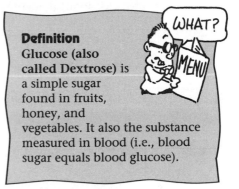

Definition
Glucose (also called Dextrose) is a simple sugar found in fruits, honey, and vegetables. It also the substance measured in blood (i.e., blood sugar equals blood glucose).

Another reason to choose complex carbs is the glucose created during digestion gets released into your blood more slowly. Simple carbohydrates are already broken down—they go straight into the blood all at once, resulting in what is unofficially known as the sugar rush, whereas complex carbohydrates are larger molecules that must be broken down. As your body processes complex carbos, small glucose molecules are released into the blood over an extended period of time—not all at once. This helps to regulate blood sugar levels, especially in people who may have problems with their blood sugars (e.g., hyperglycemia, hypoglycemia, diabetes mellitus).

Definitions

Hyperglycemia: A condition in which a person has an abnormally high blood-glucose (blood-sugar) concentration. *Hyper* means "too much", *glyce* means "glucose", *emia* means "in the blood".

Hypoglycemia: A condition characterized by a blood-sugar concentration that's abnormally low. Here, *hypo* means "too little."

Diabetes mellitus: A disorder of blood-sugar regulation usually caused by the body's insufficiency to either produce enough insulin or use it effectively.

How Much Carbohydrate Should You Eat?

As mentioned earlier, 55–60 percent of your total food for the day should consist of carbohydrate, specifically complex carbohydrate. In fact, 80 percent or more of your total carbohydrate intake should come from complex carbs and naturally-occurring sugars found in fruits and vegetables.

So what exactly does this mean in terms of food? You'll need to fill about 55–60 percent of your plate at each meal with some of these carbohydrate rich foods. Remember, don't get nit-picky about percentages. Take the easy way out and eyeball your meal selections.

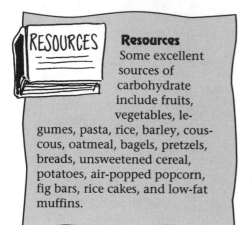

Resources
Some excellent sources of carbohydrate include fruits, vegetables, legumes, pasta, rice, barley, couscous, oatmeal, bagels, pretzels, breads, unsweetened cereal, potatoes, air-popped popcorn, fig bars, rice cakes, and low-fat muffins.

Instead of the typical bacon and eggs for breakfast, boost your carbohydrate intake with cereals, waffles, pancakes, oatmeal, or bagels. For lunch eat vegetable soups, salads with beans, whole-grain breads, pasta salads, and fresh fruit. With dinner include plenty of rice, couscous, pasta, vegetables, legumes, and all types of potatoes (go easy on the fried ones though). The idea is to have *larger* amounts of carbohydrates and much *smaller* amounts of protein and fat!

Note: in extremely rare instances, due to medical conditions such as diabetes, some people cannot tolerate these recommended carbohydrate amounts and should be under a doctor's supervision for dietary guidance.

Wanna get more specific? What's the amount of carbohydrate you need?

Formula   1. Take your total calories for the day

2. Multiply by .55–.60 (or 55 percent–60 percent)
   (this will give you a range of carbohydrate calories)

3. Divide by 4 *(this will convert your range of carbohydrate calories into grams, since 1 gram carbohydrate = 4 carbohydrate calories)*

Diet Calories	Cals from Carbs	Grams of Carbs
1600 cals =	880–960	220–240
1800 cals =	990–1080	248–270
2200 cals =	1210–1320	303–330
2800 cals =	1540–1680	385–420

The amount of carbohydrate grams remains proportional to your caloric requirements. The more calories you require, the greater amount of carbohydrates you need to eat.

Way to Go!

Make sure to include the following "forgotten" grains in your diet:

Couscous: A staple in Mediterranean countries, it is one of the easiest grains to cook, and can be found in many grocery stores.

Quinoa (pronounced "keen-wah"): It is high in protein, calcium, and iron. A native South American grain which is good in puddings, soup, and stir-fry.

Barley: Good in soups, stews, side dishes, puddings, and cereals. Found in grocery stores and available as "pot" or "scotch barley."

Millet: Available in health food stores. It is good as a side dish or stuffing for poultry. High in phosphorus and B vitamins.

Wild rice: This pseudo-grain is really a grass seed. It is high in protein and a good source of B vitamins.

Amaranath: High in protein, iron and calcium. From South America and available in health food stores and some upscale grocery stores. Serves as a good side dish or cereal.

Wheat berries: Found in most grocery stores and health food stores, it serves as a good, high-fiber cereal or substitute for rice.

Do Pasta and Other Carbohydrates Make You Fat?

One day you hear you should load up on carbs, and the next day a friend claims that pasta will make you fat. Ever feel like a nutrition yo-yo? What gives?

The story is that bread, pasta, and all other complex carbohydrates supply primo quality calories and should be included in every healthful food plan. So why all the confusion? Well for starters, some people confuse weight-gain from fat with weight-gain from carbohydrates. One gram of fat has more than double the amount of calories as one gram of carbohydrate. And what some people don't realize is that fat usually accompanies carbohydrates at a meal. For instance, people remember that they had pasta for dinner but forget that the pasta was swimming in oil, butter, cheese or alfredo sauce. Clearly the culprit for weight gain was the fat (butter, oil etc.) not the carbohydrate (pasta).

Another example is many a New Yorker's favorite staple—the bagel. Alone, a bagel is a wonderful complex carbohydrate. Add all that butter or cream cheese, and you'll wind up with a lot more calories and fat than you bargained for. The next time you question whether pasta or other carbos make you fat, think again. It's more likely the fat that is making you fat.

Carbo-Addicts Beware

There are of course some exception. We call them the "Carbo-Addicts." These people go way overboard on the starchy carbs and can, in fact, gain weight. Do you eat three bagels for breakfast, a loaf of bread for lunch, a family-sized bag of pretzels for snack, only to polish off two buckets of pasta at dinner? Hey! Watching *Monday Night Football* doesn't require carbo-loading! Unless you're actually playing the game, you're eating way too many carbs, specifically those which are denser in calories, unlike those found in fruits and vegetables. With this daily food intake, it's likely you've taken in more carbohydrates and calories than your body requires.

Remember, to maintain an ideal weight, you need that balance of "calories in equals calories out." It does not make a difference if those extra calories come from carbohydrate, protein, or fat. *Excessive calories will be stored by your body as fat.* I'm not saying that carbohydrates are fattening. Simply put, almost anything consistently overeaten can put on the pounds.

To Artificially Sweeten or Not?

Before you tear open your gazillionth non-sugar packet, read the following and learn the facts.

To date, artificial sweeteners remain the subject of much controversy. The first sugar substitute to receive US Food and Drug Administration (FDA) approval was saccharin (Sweet & Low®), and it continues to be a popular sweetener today. Although several studies have suggested that saccharin in large quantities can cause cancer (specifically bladder tumors) in laboratory rats, there have been no harmful effects shown in humans.

Another popular artificial sweetener is aspartame, better known as Nutrasweet® or Equal®. Aspartame is comprised of two protein fragments (phenylalanine and aspartic acid) and has had FDA approval since 1981. It is presently found in over 5000 different products to date, and there is no evidence of any harmful effects from its use. However, since aspartame does contain phenylalanine, individuals with the metabolic disorder PKU (an inherited disease in which the body cannot dispose of excess phenylalanine) should consult with their physician before using this sweetener.

The most recent artificial sweetener to come into the market is called acesulfame K. This FDA approved sweetener is sold under the brand name Sunett™, and to date, studies have shown it to be perfectly safe for human consumption.

Why Do People Use Artificial Sweeteners?

One reason why people use artificial sweeteners may revolve around their medical conditions. For example, sugar substitutes can be a great tool for diabetics. As noted earlier, people with diabetes cannot tolerate *real* sugar because their body is unable to produce the hormone insulin. Insulin is responsible for taking the sugar out of our blood and bringing it into our cells, where we utilize it as energy. When your body doesn't get enough insulin, sugar builds up in the blood and is unable to get into the cells. This condition is known as high blood-sugar and can be extremely dangerous for people with diabetes. Since sugar substitutes do not contain any glucose (and therefore do not require insulin), they can be effective sweeteners for people with diabetes.

A more popular reason for using artificial sweeteners is saving calories. However, this notion may not be as effective as you think! While it is true that diet soft drinks and other artificially sweetened foods can save you a lot of sugar calories, several studies have shown that people who "save calories" with these diet foods, usually wind up eating those saved calories at a later point in the day. Pretty ironic, huh? Other studies suggest that artificial sweeteners may, in fact, make you hungrier. What do you know, it may actually work to your advantage to eat the real McCoy once in a while. By the way, a real sugar packet only has 16 calories. You can burn that off walking an extra flight of stairs. Certainly something to think about the next time you grab for artificial sweetener.

The bottom line is that artificial sweeteners can safely be part of a well-balanced diet. Just don't get so carried away that you view sugar as the enemy. Remember, dietary guidelines suggest eating real sugar *in moderation*, not avoiding it altogether.

The Least You Need to Know

➤ Fifty-five to sixty percent of your total food for the day should come from carbohydrate (mostly complex carbohydrate). Foods rich in carbohydrates to include are vegetables, legumes, bread, cereal, rice, pasta, and all other grain products.

➤ Limit your intake of candy, cola, and other sugary sweets. Although they are carbohydrates, simple sugars provide you with nothing more than "simply sugar".

➤ Fruit and fruit juices are the exception to the "simple sugar" rule. Although considered simple carbohydrates, they provide a variety of important nutrients.

➤ Although carbs aren't fattening, almost anything consistently overeaten will put on the pounds—including carbohydrates.

➤ In moderation, artificial sweeteners can be an effective sugar substitute for people with diabetes mellitus, and part of a well-balanced diet for the general population. The choice between sugar and substitutes is yours.

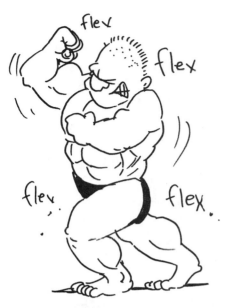

Chapter 3

Protein Power

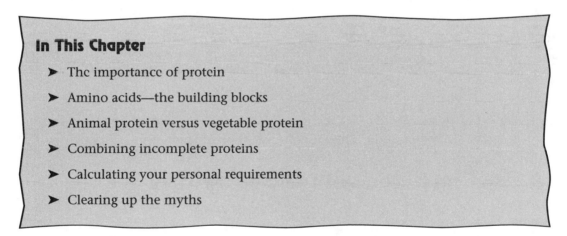

In This Chapter

➤ The importance of protein

➤ Amino acids—the building blocks

➤ Animal protein versus vegetable protein

➤ Combining incomplete proteins

➤ Calculating your personal requirements

➤ Clearing up the myths

These days, every magazine you flip through has something to say about carbohydrates and fat. Phrases like, "load up on carbs" or "eat less fat" are seemingly everywhere. Finally, it's time to learn the profile on protein—one incredibly versatile molecule. Almost everyone seems to have a basic idea of which foods are rich in protein, but do you actually know your personal requirements or understand why protein is important and how it works?

What's So Important About Protein?

First, let's point out that protein is not just in food, it is floating around *all over* your body. Did you know that your bones, organs, tendons, ligaments, muscle, cartilage, hair, nails, teeth, and skin are all made up of protein? And that's just the beginning. *Working proteins* are busy performing specific tasks in your body. These include:

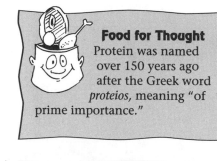

Food for Thought
Protein was named over 150 years ago after the Greek word *proteios*, meaning "of prime importance."

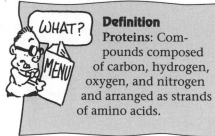

Definition
Proteins: Compounds composed of carbon, hydrogen, oxygen, and nitrogen and arranged as strands of amino acids.

➤ **Enzymes**—Proteins that facilitate and accelerate chemical reactions. Also known as protein catalysts. Each enzyme has a specific function to perform in the body.

➤ **Antibodies**—Proteins that help fight illness and disease. They are found in red blood cells.

➤ **Hemoglobin**—Proteins that transport oxygen all over the body.

➤ **Hormones (most)**—Proteins that regulate many body functions. Hormones signal enzymes to do their job, such as equalizing blood sugar levels, insulin levels, and growth.

➤ **Growth and maintenance proteins**—Proteins that serve as building materials for the growth and repair of body tissues.

The list is endless! But, I promise not to give you déjà vu of high school biology class. Besides, I'd like you to stay awake for the rest of the chapter.

A Brief Interlude with Chemistry 101

Amino acids building a protein.

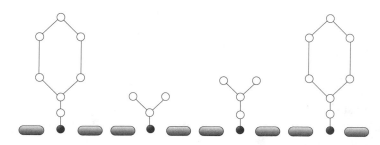

Protein is composed of carbon, hydrogen, oxygen, and nitrogen. The addition of nitrogen gives protein its unique distinction from carbohydrate and fat, along with establishing the signature name, amino acid. Much like simple sugars, which link together to form a *complex* carbohydrate (Chapter 2), amino acids are the building blocks for the more complicated protein molecule.

Amino Acids: The Building Blocks of Protein

There are a total of 20 different amino acids , and depending upon the sequence in which they appear, a specific job or function is carried out in your body. Think of amino acids as similar to the alphabet—a total of 26 letters that can be arranged in a million different ways. These arranged letters create words, which then translate into an entire language. The arrangement of amino acids is your body's "protein language," which dictates the exact tasks that need to be carried out. Therefore, proteins that make up your enzymes will have one sequence, while those that form your muscles will have a completely different one.

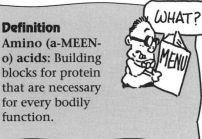

Definition
Amino (a-MEEN-o) acids: Building blocks for protein that are necessary for every bodily function.

Your Bod: The Amino Acid Recycling Bin

How does your body continually get all of the amino acids that it needs to properly function? From your body's own amino acid pool, and from eating a diet that meets your daily protein requirements. After you eat a food that contains protein, your body goes to work, breaking it down into various amino acids (different foods yield different amino acids). When the protein is completely dissected, your body absorbs the amino acids (resulting from your digested food) and rebuilds them into the sequence that you need for a specific body task. Sort of like a recycling bin!

Let's take this amino acid talk a bit further (I promise we are still in Chem 101). Out of 20 amino acids, 11 can actually be manufactured within your body. However, that means nine cannot be manufactured. You cannot function without each and every amino acid. It is "essential" that you get these nine from outside food sources. Therefore, they are appropriately called *"essential amino acids."*

Definition
Essential amino acids: Amino acids that cannot be synthesized by the body. We must get these from outside food sources.

Table 3.1 Amino Acids

Essential Amino Acids	Nonessential Amino Acids
Histidine	Glycine
Isoleucine	Glutamic Acid

continues

Table 3.1 Continued

Essential Amino Acids	Nonessential Amino Acids
Leucine	Arginine
Lysine	Aspartic Acid
Methionine	Proline
Phenylalanine	Alanine
Threonine	Serine
Tryptophan	Tyrosine
Valine	Cysteine
	Asparagine
	Glutamine

Animal Protein versus Vegetable Protein

In general, animal proteins including meat, fish, poultry, milk, cheese, and eggs are considered to be good sources of *complete proteins*. Complete proteins contain ample amounts of all essential amino acids.

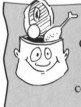

Food for Thought
Gelatin is the only animal protein that is not considered a complete protein.

Definition
Complementary proteins: Two incomplete proteins in a food that compensate for one another's shortfalls when combined.

On the other hand, vegetable proteins (grains, legumes, nuts, seeds, and other vegetables) are *incomplete proteins* because they are missing, or do not have enough of, one or more of the essential amino acids.

You Wouldn't Leave a Protein Incomplete, Would You?

So vegetable proteins are incomplete. It's really not such a big deal! You already know that grains and legumes are rich in complex carbohydrate and fiber. Now you learn that they can be an excellent source of protein as well; it just takes a little bit of work and know-how. By combining foods from two or more of the following columns—Voilà, you create a self-made complete protein. You see, the foods in one column may be missing amino acids that are present in the foods listed in another column. When eaten in combination, your body receives all nine essential amino acids.

The following are vegetable proteins that can be combined to make complete proteins.

Table 3.2 Sources of Complementary Proteins

Grains	Legumes	Nuts/Seeds
barley	beans	sesame seeds
bulgur	lentils	sunflower seeds
cornmeal	dried peas	walnuts
oats	peanuts	cashews
buckwheat	chickpeas	pumpkin
rice	soy products	other nuts
pasta		
rye		
wheat		

Table 3.3 Combinations to Create Complete Proteins

Combine Grains and Legumes	Combine Grains and Nuts/Seeds	Combine Legumes and Nuts/Seeds
peanut butter on whole-wheat bread	whole-wheat bun with sesame seeds	humus (chickpeas and sesame paste)
rice and beans	breadsticks rolled with sesame seeds	trail mix (peanuts and sunflower seeds)
bean soup and a roll	rice cakes with peanut butter	
salad with chickpeas and cornbread		
tofu-vegetable stir-fry over rice or pasta		
vegetarian chili with bread		

Also, by adding small amounts of animal protein (meat, eggs, milk, or cheese) to any of the groups, you create a complete protein. For example:

➤ oatmeal with milk

➤ macaroni and cheese

➤ casserole with a small amount of meat

➤ salad with beans and a hard cooked egg

➤ yogurt with granola

➤ bean and cheese burrito

Calculating Your Personal Protein Requirements

The amount of protein that most people need is between 10–15% of the total calories for the day, with needs being the highest for growing children and pregnant or lactating women. Since protein is abundant in a variety of foods, most people don't have to worry about not getting this required amount. However, it's quite simple to calculate your personal protein needs if you'd like to get an idea of how much you should be eating each day.

Guidelines for ages 19 years and older:

Formula:

➤ Consume 0.36 grams protein per pound of ideal body weight per day

➤ Find your body weight (or what you should weigh, if you are overweight)

➤ Multiply by 0.36 to get your daily protein requirement

Food for Thought
Keep in mind that pregnant or lactating women have the greatest protein requirements. Pregnant women need an additional 10 grams of protein a day, while breast-feeding women need 12–15 extra grams a day for the first six months.

Example:

➤ Weight = 130 pounds

➤ 130 pounds × 0.36 grams = 47 grams protein/day

To go even further, let's convert 47 grams of protein into protein calories:

➤ One gram protein = 4 calories

➤ 47 grams protein × 4 = 188 protein calories

This would be about 10% of calories from protein on a 1,800 calorie food plan.

➤ 1,800 cals × .10 = 180. Pretty close to the 188 protein cals in the above example.

Protein for the Day in a Blink of an Eye

The previous calculation gave you a number—let's see how quickly that 47 grams translates into food. The following chart lists the protein content of commonly eaten foods.

Table 3.4   Protein Content of Common Foods

Animal Proteins	Grams of Protein	Vegetable Proteins	Grams of Protein
steak, sirloin	26	peanuts (1 oz)	7
ground meat	20	walnuts (1 oz)	4
hamburger	14	peanut butter (2 T)	8
bologna	10	sesame seeds (1 oz)	5
hot dog	10	sunflower seeds (1 oz)	6
bacon (1 slice)	2	kidney beans (1/2 cup)	8
ham	21	lentils (1/2 cup)	9
turkey breast	26	chickpeas (1/2 cup)	10
roast beef	21	split peas (1/2 cup)	8
chicken, light w/o skin	26	tofu (5 oz)	10
swordfish	17	oatmeal (1 cup)	6
tuna, white, in water	25	pasta (1 cup)	7
flounder	19	brown rice (1 cup)	5
shrimp	17	white rice (1 cup)	3
cottage cheese (1/2 cup)	14	whole-wheat bread (2 slices)	5
cheddar cheese (1 oz)	7	potato, baked (small)	3
American cheese (1 oz)	6	broccoli (1/2 cup)	2
whole milk (1 cup)	8	corn (1/2 cup)	2
skim milk (1 cup)	8	spinach (1/2 cup)	3
low-fat plain yogurt (1 cup)	10	green peas (1/2 cup)	4
low-fat fruit yogurt (1 cup)	10		
egg (1)	6		

Three-ounce servings (approximately the size of a deck of cards)
Source: ©1996 First Databank

You can imagine how quickly these numbers add up, especially since most people tend to eat much more than a 3-ounce serving in one shot.

Let's take a look at a typical day.

Breakfast:

2 scrambled eggs

3 strips of bacon

2 slices of toast with margarine

glass of milk

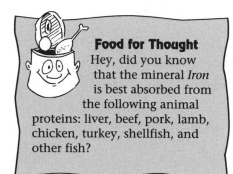

Food for Thought
Hey, did you know that the mineral *Iron* is best absorbed from the following animal proteins: liver, beef, pork, lamb, chicken, turkey, shellfish, and other fish?

Lunch:

a big fat tuna-salad sandwich (6 oz)

2 slices of bread

apple

Dinner:

steak (6-oz)

some veggies and rice

Total protein = 137 grams…YIKES!!!!

As mentioned earlier, people in industrialized countries do not have any problem meeting their protein requirements. In fact, as you can see, it's quite easy to *exceed* the amount that you actually need since our society tends to focus on meat, fish, eggs, seafood, or dairy with most every meal.

Should You Worry About Overeating Protein?

Well, maybe. The problem is that your body only utilizes what it needs. And the rest? Well, some may be used for energy, but most is just a lot of extra calories, *and usually not just protein calories.* Many of these high-protein foods are also packaged with fat; therefore, the issue of excess calories, which can ultimately translate into weight gain, can become a major concern. Furthermore, filling up on enormous portions of animal protein may crowd out grains, fruits, and veggies, which would create "macro-nutrient chaos." Remember that ultimate proportion: 55–60% carbs, 10–15% protein, <30% fat.

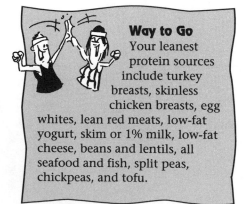

Way to Go
Your leanest protein sources include turkey breasts, skinless chicken breasts, egg whites, lean red meats, low-fat yogurt, skim or 1% milk, low-fat cheese, beans and lentils, all seafood and fish, split peas, chickpeas, and tofu.

Determine your personal protein needs and adjust your meals accordingly. You may want to prepare smaller pieces of animal protein (~3 ounces) and load a variety of veggies and grains onto your plate. Another way to tackle the situation is to mentally divide your plate into thirds with one third going to protein, starch, and vegetables.

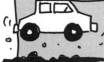

Rocky Road

Watch out for the *"high-protein"* diet, which promises quick weight loss by encouraging eating large amounts of protein while severely limiting carbohydrate intake. Sure you may lose weight, but not from any magical combination of "high protein/low carbohydrate." One reason for the weight loss may be water, because the breakdown of excessive protein causes frequent urination. Another explanation may be that your total calories are usually decreased when you're strictly limited to the high-protein foods. Think about it, how much plain protein can you really eat? Personally, I'd rather eat *one* turkey burger on a roll than *four* turkey burgers plain. Sounds both unhealthy and unappealing! What's more, the majority of people who lose weight from this type of plan usually gain it back when the carbs are reintroduced.

I do have to mention that a *small* percentage of people have a problem metabolizing carbohydrates (insulin-resistance) and therefore need to follow a high protein regimen. However, *do not* assume that you fall into this category unless diagnosed by your physician. For the majority of the population, a healthy weight loss program should include regular physical activity and a decrease in total calories from a diet rich in complex carbohydrates, moderate in protein, and low in fat.

Does Excessive Protein Build Larger Muscles?

Okay, it's time to set the record straight. It's true that protein is needed for the development of muscle, but it's not true that "extra" protein will build you bigger biceps! Body builders and other athletes do need a bit more protein than the RDA; however, this increase is already covered by the typical American diet. As mentioned earlier, we cannot store excess protein. Therefore, all those extra protein calories (and I'm sure a lot of fat went along for the ride) will most likely wind up on your...well, let's just say that I'm not talking about your quads!

In addition, anyone eating excessive protein will be urinating more frequently, since the breakdown of protein produces an increase in *urea*, a waste product in urine. You can only imagine the inconvenience of running to the bathroom every 10 minutes, let alone your risk of becoming dehydrated. Furthermore, body builders who stuff their stomachs with tremendous amounts of protein tend to skimp on carbohydrates—the key energy-providing ingredient for an optimal workout.

Q and A

Should I take amino acid supplements?

No. A well-balanced food plan (high carbs, moderate protein, and low fat), along with appropriate workouts, will be much more likely to "pump you up." Besides, megadosing can be expensive and inefficient.

The Scoop on Amino Acid Supplements

Amino acid supplements are also unnecessary. Your body only needs a certain amount of each amino acid, and most everyone receives far beyond this amount from the food they eat (both animal and vegetable protein). Although the amount that you need is vital, there is nothing "miraculous" about megadosing. In fact, overkill can be expensive and inefficient. Think about it, for next to nothing you can prepare a piece of grilled chicken with a meal instead of spending more than double for one of those "amino-acid" shakes.

The Least You Need to Know

➤ Protein is not only in food, but all over your body, performing vital functions.

➤ There are a total of 20 different amino acids that act as building blocks for the more complicated protein molecules. Nine of these amino acids must be obtained from outside food sources and are called "essential amino acids."

➤ Animal proteins are considered "complete proteins" because they contain ample amounts of all nine essential amino acids.

➤ Vegetable proteins are "incomplete proteins" since they are missing one or more of the essential amino acids. By combining two or more incomplete vegetable proteins, you can create a complete protein with all nine essential amino acids.

➤ To calculate your daily protein requirement, determine your body weight and multiple by 0.36.

➤ Some people have a tendency to go *protein overboard*, which can also mean more fat and calories, because foods high in protein may also be high in fat.

➤ Excessive protein and amino acid supplements do not build larger muscles. In fact, these myths can lead to a host of problems, including dehydration and increased fat intake.

Chapter 4

As a Matter of Fat

In This Chapter

➤ Various types of fat

➤ The heart disease connection

➤ Your cholesterol numbers and what they mean

➤ Gaining weight from excessive fat

➤ Living a low-fat lifestyle

Unless you've been living on another planet, you've heard that too much fat can create a lot of problems! Despite all of the "fat warnings" that bombard us on a daily basis, we ironically remain an overweight society that eats far too much. It's one thing to *know* what to eat (and I'm sure we would all do pretty well with a "Fat" category on *Jeopardy*), but it is an entirely different ballgame to actually make the commitment to eating healthy and then follow through with it.

And let's not forget the flip-side, low-fat does not mean no-fat! Some people take this new "low-fat religion" to radical extremes and become downright orthodox. "I'll have a broiled fish, dry, no oil; salad with mustard on the side, no dressing; steamed veggies, nothing on them; and a baked potato, plain." I guess you may as well remove your tastebuds before digging into that meal! Come on, food is supposed to be enjoyable, right?

This chapter will point out that excessive fat can lead to a host of problems including weight gain and disease. However, I would also like to emphasize to all the "fat-phobics" out there that *some* fat is perfectly okay, and with some hard work and realistic planning, everyone can find their happy medium.

Why Fat Is Fabulous

Before we begin a fat bashing session, let's investigate all of the positives on fat. Don't unclog your ears, you heard right, there are actually good things about the three letter macro-nutrient.

➤ Fat provides you with a ready source of energy.

➤ Children need fat to grow properly.

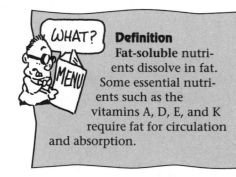

Definition
Fat-soluble nutrients dissolve in fat. Some essential nutrients such as the vitamins A, D, E, and K require fat for circulation and absorption.

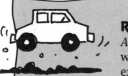

Rocky Road
All types of fat when eaten in excess can cause weight gain, but overloading on saturated fat, specifically, can also put you at risk for serious health problems, including heart disease.

➤ Fat supports the cell walls within your body.

➤ Fat enables your body to circulate, store, and absorb the fat-soluble vitamins A, D, E, and K. Without any fat you would become deficient.

➤ Fat supplies essential fatty acid that your body can't make, and must therefore get from foods.

➤ Fat helps promote healthy skin and hair.

➤ Fat makes food taste better by adding flavor, texture, and aroma.

➤ Fat provides a layer of insulation just beneath the skin. People who are extremely thin are often cold because they lack this layer of subcutaneous fat. Overweight people tend to have too much of this insulation, and become uncomfortably warm in hot weather.

➤ Fat surrounds your vital organs for protection and support. Ever wonder why your heart and kidneys aren't bouncing up and down when you go horseback riding?

Are All Fats Created Equal?

If life could only be that simple! Fat comes in a variety of packages; some are more harmful than others. In addition to watching your total fat intake, you must also pay attention to the *type* of fat you take in. Let's start from the beginning and figure out what's what in the world of fat.

Mini Glossary of Fats

The following section includes all the "fat vocabulary" you will ever need in order to speak like an expert at your next social function.

Triglyceride: The general term used for the main form of fat found in food. The structure of a TG (that's my fat slang for Triglyceride), is a *glycerol* (carbon atoms linked together) + three fatty acids. There are several Triglyceride categories, and depending upon the fatty acid composition, a TG will be classified as saturated, monounsaturated or polyunsaturated.

You may also hear about your "Triglyceride level" when the doctor takes your blood. That's because TG's, like cholesterol, are a storage form of fat in your body—circulating in the bloodstream and deposited in adipose tissue (better known as flub).

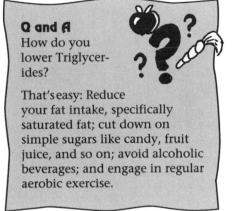

Q and A

How do you lower Triglycer- ides?

That's easy: Reduce your fat intake, specifically saturated fat; cut down on simple sugars like candy, fruit juice, and so on; avoid alcoholic beverages; and engage in regular aerobic exercise.

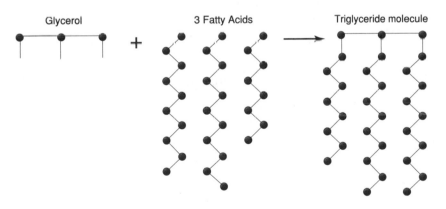

Glycerol + 3 Fatty Acids → Triglyceride molecule

Basic types of fat.

Monounsaturated fats: As mentioned above, the molecular composition of a Triglyceride can vary. When one double carbon bond is present in the fatty acid molecule (c=c) the fat is grouped as "monounsaturated" (one spot that is *not* saturated). Olive oils, peanut oils, sesame seed oils, canola oils, and avocados are high in monounsaturated fat. According to studies, these fats may help to lower blood cholesterol. But go easy with that olive oil if your weight is an issue. This "good" fat is still loaded with fat calories!

Polyunsaturated fats: Another type of unsaturated fat is polyunsaturated. Where a "mono" has 1 double carbon bond, the "poly" fat has several (c=c=c, several spots that are *not* saturated). Corn oils, cotton seed oils, safflower oils, sunflower oils, soybean oils, and mayonnaise are all predominant in polyunsaturated fat. The fat in fish is also polyunsaturated (a type called omega-3 fatty acids). Didn't think fish had any fat? Well it does (especially mackerel, salmon, albacore tuna, and sardines), but much less than most meats. What's more, the poly-fats have also been shown to help reduce the risk of heart disease. So fish away—just don't fry it!

Saturated fats: When Triglyceride molecules contain only single carbon bonds (c-c-c, unlike the double bonds you saw in mono and polyunsaturated, c=c), the fat is grouped as "saturated." Saturated fats are the demons of all fats since they are able to raise your blood cholesterol, which, in turn, can lead to heart disease. Hard to believe that a simple molecular change can make such a difference, but it can, and these guys are destructive! Animal fats found in meat, poultry, and whole-milk dairy products are all high in saturated fats. And although most vegetable oils are unsaturated, some "saturated" exceptions include coconut, palm, and palm kernel oils (found in cookies, crackers, nondairy creamers, and other baked products). Do your body a favor, make a concerted effort to cut back on these fats. You'll help protect yourself from heart disease, certain cancers, and other potential health problems.

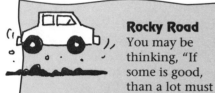

Rocky Road
You may be thinking, "If some is good, than a lot must be better." This is not necessarily the case when speaking of the fish oil supplements. Evidence is sketchy so far and no one should be popping them without a physician's approval.

Saturated, Monounsaturated, and Polyunsaturated Fats.

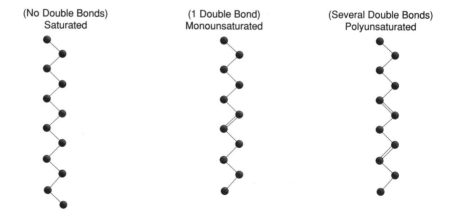

Trans-fatty acids: This type of fat is *not* naturally occurring, but created when innocent unsaturated fats undergo a manufacturing process called hydrogenation. Hydrogenation is when a liquid or semi-soft fat is transformed into a more solid state. Trans-fatty acids can become quite harmful, since they act like saturated fats inside the body and raise blood cholesterol.

So why mess with a good thing and "hydrogenate"? Because the process can help preserve food and can enable a food company to change the texture of a product. For example, margarine in the liquid form is unsaturated, but with some hydrogenation it becomes semi-soft (tub margarine). With further hydrogenation it becomes hard (stick margarine). Unfortunately, most people prefer tub and stick over liquid margarines, and end up paying the "trans-fatty" penalty. Other trans-fatty culprits include "partially hydrogenated" vegetable oils, commonly found in cakes, crackers, cookies and other baked goods. If you ever read the ingredients listed on food products, you'll know that trans-fats are everywhere.

So what can you do? It would be almost impossible to avoid trans-fat completely. Reducing your total fat and limiting the products that contain partially hydrogenated oils can significantly reduce the intake of trans-fatty acids.

Q and A

Is it better to use butter or margarine?

Butter is loaded with saturated fat, margarine is packed with trans-fatty acids. Which one do you choose? While both contain artery clogging fat, a serving of butter contains *more* artery clogging fat than most margarines. So give your blood vessels a break and spread on the margarine (specifically soft tub over stick). Better still, go all the way and buy *reduced-fat* tub spreads. You will save yourself both fat and calories.

And for all you die-hard butter fans…well, just take it easy with that knife.

Table 4.1 Most Fats Contain Combinations of All Three Types of Fat, But Are Predominantly One Type.

Saturated	Monounsaturated	Polyunsaturated
beef fat	canola oil	corn oil
butter	olive oil	cottonseed oil
whole milk	peanut oil	safflower oil
cheese	sesame oil	soybean oil
coconut oil	most nuts	sunflower oil
palm oil	avocados	margarine (soft)
palm kernel oil		mayonnaise
		fish oils
		sesame oil

The Cholesterol Connection and Heart Disease

If you have ever read a nutrition label, you know that dietary fat and cholesterol make up two very different categories. In fact, they are even measured in different units; fat is shown in grams, while cholesterol is shown in milligrams. We've already explored the facts on fat, now it's time for cholesterol.

Cholesterol is a waxy substance that contributes to the formation of many essential compounds, including vitamin D, bile acid, estrogen, and testosterone. Just imagine, without cholesterol we would have no sex drive! At this point, you may be thinking, "Hey, for a substance that does so many great things, why can't I eat as much as I want?"

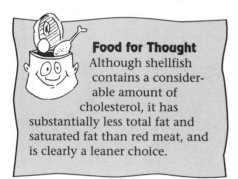

Food for Thought
Although shellfish contains a considerable amount of cholesterol, it has substantially less total fat and saturated fat than red meat, and is clearly a leaner choice.

Good question! The problem is that your liver makes all the cholesterol you'll ever need, and the unused portion all too often gets stored as plaque in your arteries.

All animal-related foods and beverages contain cholesterol, because all animals have had a liver at one time or another. Eggs, meats, fish, cheese, milk, and poultry are all sources of cholesterol. Needless to say, the slab of liver your mom ate the other night was loaded with the stuff! By the way, plant foods do not contain cholesterol, simply because they never had a liver. Makes sense, right?

Don't Be Fooled by Misleading Labels

When a label reads "no cholesterol," the food in question is not necessarily low in calories and fat. Here is a perfect example. I walked into a famous cookie store and noticed these incredibly decadent peanut butter cookies. Next to them was a sign proclaiming "NO CHOLESTEROL COOKIES." Well as far as I know, a peanut has never had a liver, and therefore peanut butter doesn't have any cholesterol! But WOW, those cookies were packed with fat. I later learned that the ingredients included peanut butter, margarine, and vegetable oil. Unfortunately, the majority of people mistook these cookies for low calorie/low-fat just because of the no-cholesterol label. I thought about screaming "Don't be conned, they're loaded with fat," but figured they would cart me away in a straight jacket. The moral of the story is simple to grasp: Next time you grab for something that reads "no cholesterol," check out the fat content; it may not be all it's cracked up to be.

So how does saturated fat work its way into the cholesterol picture? Mentioned earlier, this artery clogging culprit can also raise blood cholesterol levels. Talk about adding insult to injury, the high-fat animal foods that contain saturated fats (e.g., marbled red meats and whole-milk dairy products) provide a double-whammy because you get hit with both dietary cholesterol and saturated fat.

Table 4.2 Total fat, Saturated Fat, and the Cholesterol Content of Common Foods

Food Name	Portion	Total Fat (gr)	Saturated Fat (gr)	Cholesterol (mg)
Ground Beef, med-fat	3 oz.	17.7	6.9	76
Ground Beef, lean	3 oz.	15.7	6.2	74
Frankfurter	3 oz.	24.8	9.1	43
Chicken Breast, no skin	3 oz.	3.0	0.9	72
Turkey Breast, no skin	3 oz.	1.0	0.2	71
Liver, braised	3 oz.	4.2	1.6	331
Sole / Flounder	3 oz.	1.3	0.3	58
Swordfish	3 oz.	4.4	1.2	43
Salmon, Atlantic	3 oz.	6.9	1	60
Whole Egg	1	5.0	1.6	213
Egg Yolk	1	5.0	1.6	213
Egg White	1	0.0	0.0	0
Whole Milk	1 cup	8.1	5.1	33
Skim Milk	1 cup	0.4	0.3	4
Cheddar Cheese	1 oz.	9.4	6.0	30
American Cheese	1 oz.	8.8	5.6	27
Mozzarella / Skim Milk	1 oz.	4.5	2.9	16
Nuts	1 oz.	14.1	2.0	0
Butter	1 Tbs.	11.4	7.1	31
Margarine	1 Tbs.	11.4	2.1	0
Margarine, Red. Fat	1 Tbs.	5.7	1.0	0
Olive Oil	1 Tbs.	13.5	1.8	0

Source: ©First Databank

Your Cholesterol Report Card

YIKES! The doctor just sent you a report indicating that your blood cholesterol level is high. Are you now at risk for heart disease?

Although it's certainly not in your favor to have clogged arteries, before you write yourself off and give away all of your prized possessions, know that most people have tremendous control over lowering their numbers. Limiting the fats and oils in your diet, increasing foods rich in soluble fiber, losing weight if you're overweight, and becoming more physically active will get you headed in the right "heart-smart" direction.

Food for Thought
Some people are born with a genetic predisposition to having high cholesterol, and therefore may need the assistance of cholesterol-lowering medication.

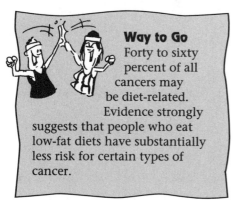

Way to Go
Forty to sixty percent of all cancers may be diet-related. Evidence strongly suggests that people who eat low-fat diets have substantially less risk for certain types of cancer.

And what do those numbers on the report card mean anyway?

Total Blood Cholesterol: This number refers to the amount of cholesterol circulating in the bloodstream, and provides a direct correlation to the amount of plaque deposited in your arteries. It is a combination of both types of cholesterol—HDL (good) and LDL (bad). Total cholesterol levels less than 200mg/dL are considered desirable. To help remember which "DL" is which, just remember this: "L" in LDL stands for "Lousy," while "H" in HDL stands for "Helpful."

HDL: The "good guys" actually help your body get rid of the cholesterol in your blood (sort of like garbage men clearing out the garbage). Thus, the higher your HDL-cholesterol number, the better off you are. An HDL-cholesterol less than 35mg/dL is considered low and increases your risk for heart disease.

LDL: The "bad guys" cause the cholesterol to build up in the walls of your arteries. Thus, the higher your LDL-cholesterol number, the greater your risk for heart disease. Desirable LDL-cholesterol is less than 130mg/dL.

Getting Fat from Eating Fat

The consequence from eating excessive fat is one that most of us know all too well, *weight gain*. Gram for gram, fat delivers more than twice the amount of calories as carbohydrate and protein. In other words, high-fat foods (e.g., meats and whole-milk dairy products) are more calorically dense than low-fat foods (e.g., grains, fruits, and veggies) and boy, those fat calories can add up quickly. A measly chocolate bar contains 240 calories; by contrast, so does an entire plateful of low-fat foods such as an apple, a banana, and a handful of pretzels. There is no comparison; you get a lot more quantity for the same amount of calories when you go low-fat. Sure, the candy bar may sound more appealing, but consider the other fats you may have consumed that same day: salad dressings, fried foods, whole-milk dairy, and fatty meats. That's a lot of fat, which means a tremendous amount of calories.

Don't get me wrong, no one should deprive themselves of the things they love (unless of course it's fried porkskins—yuck!). Like money, though, your fat needs to be strategically budgeted so you don't go overboard by the end of the day. In this case, consistently going over your budget won't leave you broke, but it will leave you fat.

Filling up on fatty foods may also crowd out the healthy stuff that keeps us fit. Great, now you're chubby and malnourished! Believe me, I'm a fellow sympathizer. It's tough with all those delicious donuts, cakes, and gooey, chocolatey treats staring you in the face all the time. And I'm certainly not one of those "genetic lean machines" who can eat whatever they want and not gain an ounce (hate every one of them!). So for most people, maintaining an ideal weight means watching total fat intake.

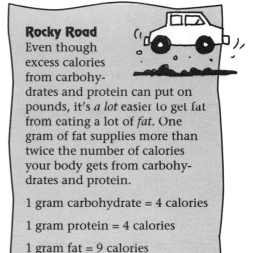

Rocky Road
Even though excess calories from carbohydrates and protein can put on pounds, it's *a lot* easier to get fat from eating a lot of *fat*. One gram of fat supplies more than twice the number of calories your body gets from carbohydrates and protein.

1 gram carbohydrate = 4 calories

1 gram protein = 4 calories

1 gram fat = 9 calories

How Much Fat and Cholesterol Should We Eat?

The American Heart Association recommends the following:

➤ Less than 30% of the day's total calories should come from fat

➤ Less than 10% of the day's total calories should come from saturated fat

➤ Less than 300 milligrams of dietary cholesterol a day

Table 4.3   A Guide to Recommended Daily Fat Intake

Daily Calories	Fat Calories	Total Fat Grams	Saturated Fat Grams
1,200	<360	<40	<13
1,500	<450	<50	<17

continues

Table 4.3 Continued

Daily Calories	Fat Calories	Total Fat Grams	Saturated Fat Grams
1,800	<540	<60	<20
2,000	<600	<67	<22
2,500	<750	<83	<28
2,800	<840	<93	<31
3,000	<900	<100	<33

Some Fats Are Easier to Spot than Others

While some fats and oils are rather obvious, others are hidden deep within our food. Take a look!

Visible fats: *butter, *cream cheese, *lard, *sour cream, mayonnaise, oil-based salad dressings, *cream or cheese based salad dressings, *animal shortenings, guacamole, cooking oils, peanut butter, and margarine.

Invisible fats: *whole-milk dairy, *high-fat meats (including bologna, pepperoni, sausage, bacon, pastrami, spare-ribs, hot dogs), *doughnuts, *cakes, *cookies, nuts, *candy bars, *chocolate chips, avocado, *ice cream, fried foods, *pizza, cole slaw, macaroni salad, and potato salad.

*Contains saturated fat

Life After Fat: Tips to Reduce the Fat in Your Diet

Get ready for a low-fat lifestyle. Read through and memorize the following suggestions for slicing off the fat without a knife.

➤ Choose low-fat dairy products whenever possible: skim or 1% milk, low-fat cheese and yogurts, low-fat sour creams, and reduced-fat ice cream.

➤ Prepare foods by roasting, baking, broiling, boiling, steaming, lightly stir-frying, or grilling. Do not fry!

➤ Remove all skin from poultry and trim all visible fat from meats.

➤ Limit your intake of red meats and try to completely avoid the higher-fat selections including salami, bologna, sausage, pepperoni, bacon, and hot dogs.

➤ Buy reduced-fat versions of margarine, butter, mayonnaise, and cream cheese.

➤ Buy low-fat salad dressings, or make your own by mixing balsamic vinegar, lots of spices, and a drop of olive oil.

➤ Instead of using butter and oily sauces, flavor your vegetables with herbs and seasonings. Also try lemon juice, spicy mustard, salsa, and flavored vinegars.

➤ Watch out for pastas swimming in oil and cream sauce. Instead, substitute marinara or other tomato-based sauces.

➤ Opt for egg white omelets (or egg substitutes) rather than whole eggs with yolk. If you can't live without eating whole eggs, limit yourself to three to four yolks per week.

➤ Pass on the ice cream, chips, and cookies. Instead snack on pretzels, fig bars, fresh fruit, and frozen yogurt.

➤ Use extra lean ground turkey breast instead of ground beef in your favorite recipes.

The "Fat-Phobic" Generation

Sure a low-fat lifestyle is the way to go, but some misinterpret this message and become utterly neurotic. Are you afraid to even touch anything that may have at one time possibly come in contact with fat? When ordering in a restaurant, do you create such chaos that your waiter is off and running to his or her shrink?

It may sound funny, but it's no laughing matter to be completely preoccupied with fat. Certainly a low-fat diet is an essential part of being healthy; however, taking this concept to radical extremes can place incredible restraints on social eating, let alone set you up for a more serious eating disorder. If your reasoning is weight control, think again! Some fat is fine, and I promise that you can maintain your ideal body weight (a reasonable weight of course), while allowing yourself to enjoy foods with fat every once in a while.

In fact, joining a "fat-free cult" doesn't necessarily mean that you automatically lose weight. Quite frequently I come across clients who cannot seem to drop an aggravating 5-10 pounds—even while following a strictly fat-free regimen. How can that be?

The answer is rather obvious: They simply overcompensate with the fat-free products. For the most part, the explosion of lower-fat foods on the market has been a wonderful tool, enabling people to painlessly lower their cholesterol and total fat intakes. Unfortunately for some people, the word "low-fat" means carte-blanche to eating huge amounts. Just because a product is fat-free doesn't mean it's calorie-free. As a matter of fact, many lower-fat foods can pack in just as many calories as their original fat-containing counterparts.

Do you have a friend who will not go near a "real" chocolate chip cookie, but doesn't hesitate to inhale an entire box of the fat-free version? Which is worse, the cookie with fat at 75 calories, or 15 no-fat cookies at a whopping 750 calories? You've heard it a million times, no matter where they come from, calories still count in the battle of the bulge.

Overly preoccupied with fat? Relax, take a deep breath and splurge every now and then. I promise you won't explode!

The Least You Need to Know

➤ Fats perform vital roles in the body including providing stored energy, storing and circulating fat-soluble vitamins, and providing a layer of insulation underneath the skin.

➤ The three types of fat include monounsaturated, polyunsaturated, and saturated.

➤ All types of fat, when eaten in excess, can cause a variety of health problems including weight gain.

➤ Saturated fat has the destructive capability to increase blood cholesterol and therefore promote heart disease.

➤ The American Heart Association recommends less than 30% of daily calories come from total fat, less than 10% of daily calories come from saturated fat, and less than 300 milligrams of dietary cholesterol be consumed each day.

➤ Live a "low-fat lifestyle" by limiting your intake of red meat, whole-milk dairy, fried foods, high-fat spreads, and oily sauces. Switch to low-fat milk, yogurts, and cheese, while jazzing up foods with herbs, spices, lemon juice, and Dijon mustard.

➤ Although low-fat and fat-free foods are great for your diet, every diet must have some sort of fat in it. A totally "fat-free diet" is dangerous because fat is responsible for vital body functions.

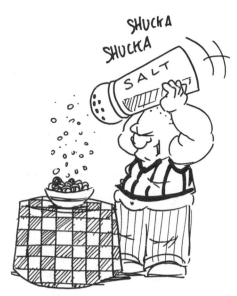

SHUCKA
SHUCKA

SALT

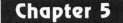

Chapter 5

Don't "As-salt" Your Body

In This Chapter

➤ What sodium can do for you

➤ Sodium and water retention

➤ The high blood pressure connection

➤ How much is recommended?

➤ Decreasing your intake

True story. I had a friend in college who would buy a large bucket of salted popcorn at the movie theater. Once in her seat, she'd whip out a salt shaker hidden in her jacket and proceed to heavily salt each individual kernel before popping it in her mouth. That's a true salt addict! A sure win for "Miss Water-Retention USA," if there should ever be such a contest. I can promise you, you'd never catch me sharing any of her popcorn; first, I was majoring in nutrition (and you never know when a professor might be sitting in the row behind), but more importantly, I couldn't stomach all that salt.

A lot of your salt influence has to do with the way you grew up and your cultural background. (Some ethnic cuisines are loaded with salty condiments and seasonings.) Were your parents into the salt shaker? Were the first three ingredients in grandma's secret recipes salt, salt, and salt? If so, you were clearly "salt corrupted" as a kid! And what about our convenience food generation? Nowadays, people are so happy to buy ready prepared, prepackaged, frozen, and microwaveable meals, they don't realize the colossal amounts of salt they cram into their bodies.

So what's the problem with a salty love affair? Using excessive amounts may lead to uncomfortable water-retention and the more serious problem of high blood pressure. Although it has been proven that *not* everyone is "salt sensitive," there is no way to tell if you might develop high blood pressure from eating too much salt. Therefore, it is certainly better to be safe than sorry when your health is at stake. Read on and learn how to give up the shakes without giving up taste!

All About Salt

Salt is composed of 40% sodium and 60% chloride. When most people speak of the problems associated with salt, they are usually referring to the part of salt called sodium. So what exactly is sodium and what does it do?

Sodium is a mineral that is essential for many important functions, such as:

➤ Controlling the fluid balance within your body

➤ Transmitting electrical nerve impulses

➤ Contracting muscles (including your heart)

➤ Absorbing nutrients across cell membranes

➤ Maintaining your body's acid/base balance

With such a wonderful resume, why worry about your sodium intake? Although sodium is an element that is essential for good health, your body requires less than $1/10$ teaspoon of salt each day. Can you imagine that the average American consumes 5–18 times more than that on a daily basis? That's one salty society we live in! In fact, most people could stand to substantially cut back.

Feeling a Bit Waterlogged?

Have your fingers ever been so swollen that it's literally impossible to get your rings on or off? Oh, the uncomfortable aftermath from excessive salt!

It's common to experience a temporary bloating or swelling after eating highly salted foods. You see, your body must have a certain balance of sodium and water at all times. Extra salt requires extra water, resulting in water-retention. Where does this extra water or fluid come from? Usually your glass. Salt triggers your thirst response as a method to balance out the sodium-water concentration. Ever wonder why you are so incredibly thirsty after munching on salty pretzels or nuts? It's not just a coincidence that all of the snacks offered in drinking establishments are covered with salt. What a strategy—the more you eat the more you drink!

Try performing this test: Record your weight one morning. Then, before going to bed that night, eat a large serving of heavily salted popcorn or other food (drink lots of water). Weigh yourself again the next morning. It is amazing how much water that salt can retain! But for all you dieters out there, remember, this is water weight—not fat weight! So don't panic—it will be gone in a couple of hours.

Note: Do not, under any circumstances, try the above test if you have any medical condition.

Can't Take the Pressure!

For reasons that are not completely understood, salt can play an active role in raising the blood pressure in people who are salt-sensitive.

What Exactly Is High Blood Pressure?

When your heart beats, it pumps blood into your arteries and creates a pressure within them. High blood pressure (also known as hypertension), is a condition that occurs when literally too much pressure is placed on the walls of the arteries. This can occur if there is an increase in blood volume, or the blood vessels themselves constrict or narrow.

People who are genetically sensitive to salt are not able to efficiently get rid of extra sodium through their urine. Therefore, that extra sodium hangs around, drawing in extra water, which means an increase in blood volume. This increased blood volume can then stimulate the vessels to constrict, creating increased pressure.

For example, imagine a garden hose with a normal flow of water running through it. Smooth sailing, no problem. Now think about the increased pressure on the hose when you drastically turn up the amount of

Resources
Although your salt intake may vary from day to day, the amount of sodium in your body doesn't generally vary by more than 2%. Your body is quite efficient at conserving sodium if you need it, or excreting it if you have a surplus.

Definition
Hyponatremia: Excessive loss of sodium and water due to persistent vomiting, diarrhea, or profuse sweating. In this case both water and salt must be replenished to maintain the correct balance for your body.

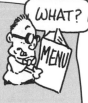

Definition
Hypertension: The medical term for sustained high blood pressure. Contrary to how this term may sound, it does not refer to being tense, nervous, or hyperactive.

water rushing out. And what if you were to pinch off spots of this hose mimicking a constricted blood vessel? A garden hose may be able to endure the wear and tear, but your arteries can become extremely damaged by such constant pressure. "How damaged?" you ask. As Billy Joel once said, "Heart-a-tack-tack-tack-tack." Let's not forget about other results, which include stroke (a brain attack) and kidney disease.

Food for Thought

➤ 1.5 million Americans suffer a heart attack every year

➤ 500,000 Americans suffer a stroke every year

Source: American Heart Association 1996

What Causes High Blood Pressure?

According to recent statistics, one out of every four American adults—nearly 60 million people—has high blood pressure. In a small percentage of people, this increased pressure is from an underlying problem such as kidney disease, or a tumor of the adrenal gland. However, in 90–95% of all cases, the cause is unclear. That's why it is known as the *"silent killer,"* it just creeps up without any warning. Whereas some of the contributing factors are *not* controllable, others can be quite controllable.

Risk factors that cannot be controlled:

➤ **Age:** The older you get, the more likely you are to develop high blood pressure. Another thing to look forward to!

➤ **Race:** African-Americans tend to have high blood pressure more often than whites. They also tend to develop it earlier and more severely.

➤ **Heredity:** High blood pressure can run in families. If you have a family history, you're twice as likely to develop it than others.

Risk factors that can be controlled are:

➤ **Obesity:** Being extremely overweight is clearly related to high blood pressure. In fact, nearly 60% of all high blood pressure cases deal with overweight patients. By losing weight—even a small amount—obese individuals can significantly reduce their blood pressure.

➤ **Sodium consumption:** Reducing the intake of salt can lower blood pressure in people who are salt sensitive.

➤ **Alcohol consumption:** Regular use of alcohol can dramatically increase blood pressure in some people. Fortunately, alcohol's effect on blood pressure is completely reversible. Limit yourself to a maximum of two drinks a day.

➤ **Smoking:** Although the long term effect of smoking on blood pressure is still unclear, the short term effect is: It can raise blood pressure briefly. However, given that both smoking and high blood pressure have been linked to heart disease, smoking compounds the risk.

➤ **Oral contraceptives:** Women who take birth control pills may develop high blood pressure.

➤ **Physical inactivity:** Lack of exercise can contribute to high blood pressure. By becoming more active with moderate exercise, an inactive person can get into better shape, feel terrific, and help keep his or her blood pressure in check.

Investigating Your Blood Pressure Numbers

Your doctor measures two numbers when checking your blood pressure, Systolic and Diastolic.

Q and A

What's the normal blood pressure reading?

Normal blood pressure readings fall within a range. It is not one set of numbers; however, it should be *less* than 140/90 if you are an adult.

WHAT? Definitions

Systolic pressure is the top, larger number. This represents the amount of pressure that is in your arteries while your heart contracts (or beats). During this contraction, blood is ejected from the heart and into the blood vessels that travel throughout your body.

Diastolic pressure is the bottom, smaller number. This represents the pressure in your arteries while your heart is relaxing between beats. During this relaxation period, your heart is filling up with blood for the next squeeze. Although both numbers are critically important, your doctor may be more concerned with an elevated diastolic number because this indicates that there is increased pressure on the artery walls even when your heart is resting.

Q and A

How do you know if you have high blood pressure?

You don't! High blood pressure is known as the "silent killer" because it has no symptoms. In fact, many people can have hypertension for years without knowing it; by that time, their body organs may have already been damaged. Stay on top of your health and have your blood pressure checked regularly by a qualified health professional.

How to Lower High Blood Pressure

If your blood pressure is high, don't panic. Most people can significantly lower their numbers with know-how and determination. A diagnosis of high blood pressure often requires reducing salt intake, losing excess weight, increasing exercise, and in some instances, taking medication.

➤ **Diet:** Lose weight if you are overweight by cutting back on calories and fat. Reduce your consumption of sodium by avoiding salty foods, and limit the amount of alcohol you drink. Better yet, avoid it completely.

➤ **Exercise:** Become physically active and plan to get some type of exercise at least four times a week. Check with your doctor before beginning any diet or exercise program.

➤ **Medication:** For some people, diet and exercise are just not enough. In this case your doctor may give you medication to help lower your blood pressure.

➤ If you smoke—QUIT!!!

How Much Sodium Is Recommended?

Many question the "one size fits all" recommendation because not everyone is "salt-sensitive." However, there is no test for salt sensitivity, therefore, it makes sense for *everyone* to play it safe and follow a prudent approach. Most health professionals recommend limiting your intake of sodium to no more than 2,400 milligrams per day. This includes both the salt you add and the sodium that is already present in foods you eat. Become familiar with the following list of high-sodium foods, and learn to balance your diet so you don't go sodium overboard. Note, if you have high blood pressure, your doctor may prescribe a more severe sodium restriction.

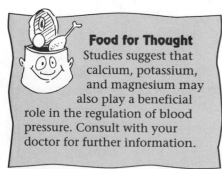

Food for Thought
Studies suggest that calcium, potassium, and magnesium may also play a beneficial role in the regulation of blood pressure. Consult with your doctor for further information.

Common Foods that Are High in Sodium

Seasonings and Cooking Aids	Portion Size	Sodium (mg)
Baking Powder	1 teaspoon	426
Baking Soda	1 teaspoon	1,259
Table Salt	1 teaspoon	2,300
Garlic Salt	1 teaspoon	2,050
Bouillon Cube, chicken	1 item	1,152
Bouillon Cube, beef	1 item	864
Monosodium Glutamate (MSG)	1 Tablespoon	1,914 mgms
Salad Dressing, italian	1 Tablespoon	116
Soy Sauce	1 Tablespoon	1,029
Low-Sodium Soy Sauce	1 Tablespoon	660
Butter Buds	1 Tablespoon	177

Canned Food Items	Portion Size	Sodium (mg)
Tuna, canned	3 ounces	303
Sardines, canned	3 ounces	261
Caviar, black & red	1 Tablespoon	240
Chicken Noodle Soup	1 cup	1,106
Vegetable Soup	1 cup	795
Veg. Beef Soup (low-sodium)	1 cup	57
Corn, canned	$1/2$ cup	266
Asparagus, canned	$1/2$ cup	472
Sauerkraut, canned	$1/2$ cup	780

Processed/Cured and Smoked Meats	Portion Size	Sodium (mg)
Bologna	3 ounces	832
Salami	3 ounces	1,922
Hot Dog	1 item	639
Smoked Turkey	3 ounces	916
Smoked Fish	3 ounces	619
Smoked Sausage	3 ounces	853

continues

continued

Snack Foods	Portion Size	Sodium (mg)
Salted Nuts	1 ounce	230
Pretzels	1 ounce	476
Corn Chips	1 ounce	164
Potato Chips	1 ounce	133
Popcorn	1 ounce	179
Saltines	5 crackers	180
Peanut Butter	1 Tablespoon	76

Dairy Products	Portion Size	Sodium (mg)
American Cheese	1 ounce	336
Cheddar Cheese	1 ounce	176
Parmesan Cheese	1 ounce	527
Cottage Cheese	1/2 cup	459
Butter	1 tablespoon	116
Margarine	1 tablespoon	132

Common Breakfast Cereals	Portions Size	Sodium (mg)
Rice Krispies	1 ounce	294
Corn Flakes	1 ounce	351
All-Bran	1 ounce	320
Cheerios	1 ounce	307
Special K	1 ounce	306
Raisin Bran	1 ounce	155

Source: ©First Databank Bowes & Church's, Food Values of Portions Commonly Used, 15th ed., 1989

Salt-Less Solutions

Giving up salt does not mean giving up the pleasure of eating. However, you will need to become a bit more selective with certain food products and much more creative in the seasoning department. The following guidelines can show you how to drastically cut the amount of salt in your food and body.

➤ Enhance the flavor of your foods with spices and herbs. Try allspice, basil, bay leaves, chives, cinnamon, curry powder, dill, garlic (not garlic salt), onion (not onion salt), rosemary, nutmeg, thyme, sage, turmeric, mace, and salt substitutes.

➤ Avoid putting a salt shaker on your breakfast, lunch, or dinner table.

➤ Choose fresh and frozen vegetables when possible (the canned versions generally contain a lot of salt). When canned is the only option, reduce the salt by draining the liquid and rinsing the vegetables in water before eating.

➤ Here I go with another plug for fresh fruit, it's naturally low in sodium!

➤ Go easy on condiments that contain considerable amounts of salt, including catsup, mustard, monosodium glutamate (MSG), salad dressings, sauces, bouillon cubes, olives, sauerkraut, and pickles. Stock your kitchen with low-sodium versions of soy sauce, teriyaki sauce, steak sauce, and anything else you may find in your travels.

➤ Select unsalted (or reduced salt) nuts, seeds, crackers, popcorn, and pretzels.

➤ Take it easy with cheese. Unfortunately, it not only has a lot of fat, but sodium as well. If you're feeling extra motivated, stock your fridge with low-salt/low-fat brands.

➤ Read labels carefully and try to choose foods lower in sodium, especially when choosing frozen dinners, canned soups, packaged mixes, and combination dishes.

➤ Beware of processed luncheon cold cuts, as well as cured and smoked meats because they are saturated with sodium. This includes bacon, bologna, salami, sausages, hot dogs, smoked turkey, fish, and beef. Also be aware that canned fish (tuna, salmon, and sardines) is extremely high in sodium.

➤ When dining in Chinese or Japanese restaurants, ask for meals without MSG or added salt. Nowadays, you can also request low-sodium soy sauce for your table. If they don't have any, dilute the regular by adding a Tablespoon of water.

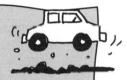

Rocky Road
Be aware that some over-the-counter medicines contain a lot of sodium. For example, a two tablet dose of dissolvable alka-seltzer (plop plop fizz fizz) has a whopping "1134 milligrams of sodium" (each single tablet provides 567 milligrams). Instead, opt for the caplets that you swallow—they *only* contain 1.8 milligrams. Quite a drastic difference.

The Least You Need to Know

➤ Salt is made up of 40% sodium and 60% chloride. The mineral sodium is essential for many important functions. It maintains body fluids, contraction of muscles, and transmits nerve impulses.

➤ Sodium and water must be in a certain balance within your body. After eating a meal with a lot of salt, your body will retain excess water. The end result is a "temporary" water retention. Don't panic, this water weight will be gone in a couple of hours.

➤ Eating a high-sodium diet can increase blood pressure in people who are "salt-sensitive."

➤ People diagnosed with high blood pressure often need to reduce their salt intake, lose excess weight, increase exercise, and in some instances, take blood pressure-lowering medication.

➤ Since salt sensitivity is *not* something we are tested for, everyone should follow a prudent approach by limiting their sodium intake to less than 2,400 milligrams per day.

➤ Reduce your sodium intake by using herbs, spices, and seasonings instead of salt. Limit canned food items, salty snack foods, luncheon cold cuts, and meats that have been smoked or cured. Go easy on high-sodium condiments such as soy sauce, teriyaki sauce, mustard, catsup, olives, pickles, and sauerkraut. Also read labels carefully and opt for the lower sodium foods.

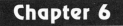

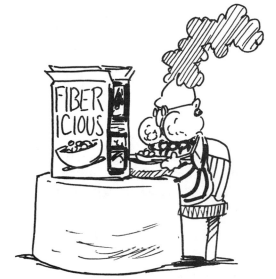

Chapter 6

Moving Right Along with Fiber

In This Chapter

➤ What is fiber?

➤ Insoluble fiber vs. soluble fiber

➤ The many benefits from a fiber-rich diet

➤ How much fiber do you need?

➤ Increasing your daily fiber intake

So, you're a little constipated? Got high cholesterol? Want to reduce your risk of colon cancer? Have I got a food for you! So what is this magical food, and where can you get some of the stuff? Well, the nice part is that you don't have to buy any special potions or formulas, or seek the advice of your local medicine man. This incredible healer is conveniently found in some of your favorite carbohydrate-rich foods.

Fiber Facts: What Is Fiber Anyway?

Fiber is a mix of many different substances found in plant cell walls is not digestible by the human body. *In it comes and out it goes.* So how can a substance we cannot even digest, (and by the way, has no nutritional value), be so beneficial? Might sound crazy, but once inside your body, fiber has been shown to do some pretty amazing things. The term *dietary fiber,* when listed on a nutrition label, simply refers to the amount of these indigestible substances in a specific food product. This way you can identify a food rich in fiber.

Soluble versus Insoluble: Let's Investigate the Difference

Fiber is broken down into two categories, insoluble and soluble, depending upon its ability to dissolve (or not dissolve) in water. Some foods contain *both* soluble and in-soluble fiber, while others are predominant in only one. The key is to eat a variety of fiber-rich foods each day and receive the beneficial effects from both types.

Soluble Fiber

Water-soluble fiber readily dissolves in water. Technically speaking, soluble fibers include pectins, gums, and mucilages. It's obvious, however, that these terms won't be of any help to you in your grocery store. So translated into "real-food" terminology, you'll find soluble fiber in the following:

➤ oats

➤ brown rice

➤ barley

➤ oat bran

➤ beans

➤ rye

➤ seeds

➤ vegetables

➤ fruits (especially apples, strawberries, oranges, bananas, nectarines, and pears)

So why all the hoopla? Well for starters, foods rich in *soluble fiber* have been shown to help decrease blood cholesterol, therefore reducing the risk of heart disease. Another benefit comes from its ability to slow the absorption of glucose (sugar in the blood), which may in turn help control blood sugar levels in diabetics.

Insoluble Fiber

Next, we have the type of fiber that does not readily dissolve in water called *water-insoluble.* Insoluble fiber includes lignin, cellulose, and hemicellulose. And once again, converted into understandable food terms, we are talking about the following:

➤ wheat bran

➤ whole-wheat breads and cereals

➤ legumes

➤ fruits

➤ vegetables

As you can see, there are some foods that are mentioned on both lists, indicating that they provide both soluble *and* insoluble fiber.

Insoluble fiber is primarily responsible for accelerating intestinal transit time, along with increasing and softening stools. In other words, insoluble fiber is responsible for "moving things along," if you know what I mean. In addition to promoting regularity, insoluble fiber has been shown to decrease your risk for colon cancer and diverticulosis.

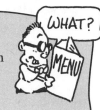

Definition
Diverticulosis: An illness or condition where tiny pouches (called diverticula) form in the wall of the colon. The condition is often without symptoms, but when the pouches become infected or inflamed, it can be painful. When this happens, the condition is known as diverticulitus, which can cause fever, abdominal pain, and diarrhea.

Reducing Your Risk of Colon Cancer

Can a diet rich in fiber actually lower your chance of developing colon cancer? Several studies say yes, and it makes perfect sense! Think about it. *Insoluble fiber* helps move waste material through your intestines more quickly. Therefore, there is less time for suspicious substances to lurk around and possibly damage your colon. In addition, fiber may bind with possibly harmful bacteria, transporting it through the intestines and out of your body. While we are down in the area, it's a perfect time to point out that softer, and more regular bowel movements can also prevent constipation and reduce your chance of getting hemorrhoids.

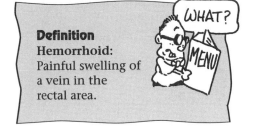

Definition
Hemorrhoid: Painful swelling of a vein in the rectal area.

Lowering Your Cholesterol Level

If your cholesterol tends to be a bit high, or you'd just like to maintain an already low number, you may want to increase your *soluble fiber*. Soluble fibers have been shown to bind with cholesterol and pull it out of the body. Fruits, vegetables, legumes, oats, and all foods made with oat-bran can therefore reduce your risk for heart and artery disease by lowering blood cholesterol. Another thought is that high-fiber foods can displace some of the high-fat, artery-clogging foods in your diet—a double impact!

Yes, You Can Feel Fuller with Less Food

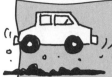

Rocky Road Just because a food sounds healthy does not necessarily mean that it is. Some **bran muffins** are loaded with fat and sugar—certainly not worth the small amount of fiber they provide.

Did you ever feel like a plate of vegetables expanded in your stomach after you ate it? Well, it did! Eating fiber-rich foods can promote feelings of fullness because they absorb water and swell inside your body. You may also feel full for a longer period of time if you choose a meal with some soluble fiber. Unlike insoluble fiber, which quickly moves food through your body, soluble fiber tends to stick around a while longer, keeping you full and satisfied.

Does this mean that you'll lose weight from eating a lot of fiber? It does if you eat these foods *instead* of the high-fat, high-calorie stuff. But eat them in addition to all the junky food, and your chance of becoming slim is, well, slim.

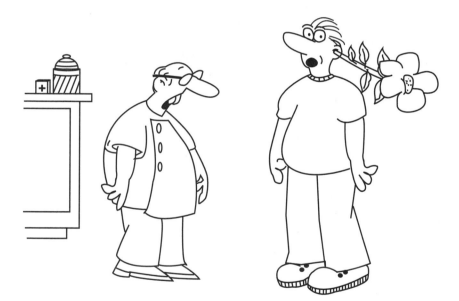

"I think you're eating too much fiber!"

How Much Fiber Do You Need?

Although there is not a Recommended Daily Amount (RDA), most leading health experts agree that we should aim for 20–35 grams of dietary fiber each day (a mix of both soluble and insoluble). Below are a few ideas to help you raise your intake of fiber.

Ready Made Menu

This sample day provides about 31 grams of fiber.

Breakfast	bowl of **bran cereal** with milk
	banana
	glass of juice
Lunch	roast beef sandwich on whole wheat bread
	cup of **vegetable barley soup**
	apple with skin
	lots of water
Snack	**chewy fruit bar**
	low-fat yogurt
Dinner	**mixed green salad**
	grilled fish with **sautéed carrots**
	baked sweet potato
	fresh strawberries
	club soda with lemon

Tips to Increase the Fiber in Your Diet

As you read the tips below, keep these points in mind. It's important to increase your fiber *gradually* (sometimes over several weeks), because your body needs time to adjust. For example, if you are a newcomer to the world of fiber, start with 20 grams each day for the first week. Increase to 25 grams per day the second week, and—if your stomach can handle it—graduate to 30+ grams per day by week three. Also, drink plenty of fluids. Fiber acts as a bulking agent by absorbing some of the fluid in your body. Extra fluids will prevent you from becoming dehydrated, and most importantly, help that bulk to move merrily on it's way!

➤ Read nutrition labels. Generally, a food considered to be a good source of fiber should have at least 2.5 grams per serving.

➤ Start your day with a high-fiber breakfast cereal. Supermarkets are flooded with them. Read the nutrition label and select a cereal that offers more than 2 grams per serving.

➤ Add a few tablespoons of wheat bran to your cereal, cottage cheese, yogurts, and salads.

➤ Include plenty of fresh or frozen vegetables in your day. Add them to soups, pizza, sandwiches, stir-frys, pastas, omelets, rice, and anything else you can think of.

➤ Eat breads and pasta made from wheat, rye, and oat products, along with brown rice, barley, and bulgur.

➤ Don't forget about fruit! Add fruit to your cereal (hot or cold), top off your pancakes and waffles with fruits, mix fruits into yogurts and salads, or simply enjoy them plain. Remember, whole fruit, with seeds and peels intact, provides more fiber than most fruit juice.

➤ Cook with beans and lentils. They are loaded with fiber. Enjoy them in soups, stews, salads, burritos, and a million other creative entrees.

➤ Get your fiber from food sources, not supplements. Food is a natural provider of not only fiber, but other essential nutrients as well.

At the end of this chapter is a handy list of foods high in fiber for you to refer to.

Don't Overdo It!

Can you ever eat too much fiber? You sure can, especially if your body is not used to it. I can remember a client who ate half a box (*large box*) of high-fiber cereal and spent the entire day doubled over in his bathroom. Overloading on fiber can cause severe bloating, cramping, gas, diarrhea, and other abdominal discomforts.

Furthermore, excessive amounts of fiber can decrease the absorption of important vitamins and minerals. With all this in mind, once again, be sure to increase your fiber *gradually,* over a period of several weeks, and drink plenty of extra fluids to help the fiber pass through your system. The key is to pay attention to your body's response so you can figure out the amount you can handle at one time.

The Least You Need to Know

➤ Fiber is the indigestible substance found in plants, and is classified under two categories: *water-soluble and water-insoluble.*

➤ Most foods contain combinations of both fibers. Foods particularly rich in soluble-fiber include oats, oat bran, legumes, rye, fruits, and vegetables. Foods rich in insoluble-fiber include wheat bran, whole wheat breads and cereals, legumes, fruits, and vegetables.

➤ Evidence suggests that *soluble* fiber can help lower blood cholesterol and improve the control of blood sugar in diabetics. Insoluble fiber has been reported to decrease the risk for colon cancer and diverticulosis, along with preventing hemorrhoids and constipation.

➤ The recommended fiber intake is 20–35 grams a day, and is an important part of every well-structured food-plan for the average adult.

➤ Increase your fiber gradually to give your body time to adjust. Also, be sure to drink plenty of extra fluids.

FRUITS	GRAMS OF FIBER
Raspberries (1 cup)	5.50
Pear (1)	4.65
Blueberries (1 cup)	4.00
Prunes (5)	3.00
Apple (1)	3.00
Orange (1)	3.00
Strawberries (1 cup)	2.70
Grapes (1 $\frac{1}{2}$ cups)	2.30
Banana (1)	2.00
Peach (1)	2.00
Grapefruit ($\frac{1}{2}$)	1.70
Nectarine (1)	1.60

VEGETABLES (all servings $\frac{1}{2}$ cup cooked)	GRAMS OF FIBER
Green Peas	4.00
Broccoli	3.60
Brussels Sprouts	3.00
Sweet Potato (small)	3.00
Baked Potato with skin (small)	2.50
Carrots	2.50
Spinach	2.20
Corn	1.70

BREADS and GRAINS	GRAMS OF FIBER
Barley (1 cup cooked)	8.80
Whole Wheat bread (2 slices)	3.20

continues

continued

BREADS and GRAINS	GRAMS OF FIBER
Brown Rice ($^3/_4$ cup cooked)	2.50
Bran Muffin (1)	2.50

CEREALS (measured by weight, therefore serving sizes will vary)	GRAMS OF FIBER
Fiber One ($^1/_2$ cup)	12.90
100% Bran ($^1/_2$ cup)	9.75
All Bran ($^1/_3$ cup)	8.40
Bran Buds ($^1/_3$ cup)	7.70
Bran Flakes ($^3/_4$ cup)	5.00
Raisin Bran ($^3/_4$ cup)	4.50
Shredded Wheat ($^3/_4$ cup)	4.00
Oatmeal ($^1/_2$ cup cooked)	2.20
Wheat Bran (4 Tablespns)	2.00
Wheat Germ (2 Tablespns)	1.50

BEANS (all servings equal $^1/_2$ cup cooked)	GRAMS OF FIBER
Pinto	6.40
Navy	4.70
White	4.40
Kidney	4.30
Black	3.60

Sources: ©1996 First Databank

Bowes & Church's Food Values of Portions Commonly Used, 15th Ed., 1989

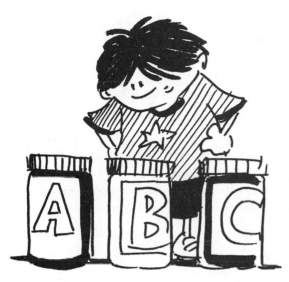

Vitamins and Minerals: The "Micro" Guys

In This Chapter

➤ What are vitamins and minerals?

➤ The RDAs and individual nutrients

➤ The role of antioxidants

What's wrong with this picture?

A woman walked into my office for an initial consult. After introducing herself, she pulled open a large duffel bag filled to the rim with vitamin and mineral bottles. "I take one of each, every day," she claimed. "Why?" I asked. "Well, a neighbor told me about extra Bs, and my hairdresser recommended extra iron, and the others I can't seem to remember."

Pretty scary stuff, but unfortunately this story is not so uncommon. Popping pills has certainly become a popular morning ritual throughout this country. And why not? We've all heard the dramatic tales of vitamins and minerals. From health food stores to infomercials, everyone seems to be buzzing about megadosing on one thing or another. Needless to say, the vitamin industry is big business, with annual sales reaching the *multi-billion dollar* level!

But do you really need all of the pills? Chances are you don't. With so much misinformation floating around, it's no wonder some people swallow exorbitant amounts of supplements they don't need. By the way, those extra supplements are literally money down the toilet because your body usually filters out the extra stuff. Talk about expensive urine! What's worse, some vitamins do not get flushed out and can potentially become toxic!

Don't get me wrong, vitamins and minerals are essential for normal functioning, and without them you could not survive. However, your body only requires minute amounts of these "micro-guys," and most nutrition experts agree that the best way to get all the vitamins and minerals you need is to eat a balanced, varied diet. While some groups of people *can* benefit from supplementation, it is important to check with a competent health professional before running out to your nearest drugstore.

Get ready to buckle in, and find out if you are getting what your body needs. This chapter will help to clear up the facts on vitamins and minerals.

What Are Vitamins and Minerals?

In previous chapters, you became familiar with the macro-nutrients carbohydrate, protein, and fat. Now it's time to understand the micro-nutrients (i.e., vitamins and minerals), which exist *within* the macro-nutrients. Although the macro-nutrients receive top billing, these micro-guys are equally important in our diets because they perform specific jobs that enable your body to operate efficiently.

Think about carbohydrate, protein, and fat as the rock stars on stage. Now imagine the vitamins and minerals as the backup singers, the band, and all of the people that help produce the concert. The big guys and little guys must work together to get the job done, with the end result being one heck of a show!

That's how your body works. You eat the carbohydrate, protein, and fat, which in turn supply your body with the 13 vitamins and at least 22 minerals you need. Although tiny in size and quantity, these nutrients accomplish the mighty tasks that keep your body going. Furthermore, a lack of any one will cause a unique deficiency that can only be corrected by supplying that particular nutrient.

The RDAs: Recommended Dietary Allowances

The Recommended Dietary Allowances (RDAs) are standards set by an expert committee known as the Food and Nutrition Board of the National Academy of Sciences/National Research Council. These recommendations list the average daily requirements for a variety of nutrients (i.e., vitamins and minerals), and are intended for healthy people. Note: People with certain illnesses may require more or less of specific nutrients. The RDA guidelines are set slightly higher than the level your body actually needs, building in a precautionary safety net.

Although the table is a good personal reference to have on hand, there is no reason for you to start calculating or memorizing these numbers. Simply eating a variety of foods from the five food groups automatically provides the levels your body requires. Don't panic if you fall short of a nutrient every once in a while—a deficiency does not develop overnight. However, you can get into trouble if you repeatedly shortchange your body of a specific vitamin or mineral.

Estimated Safe and Adequate Daily Dietary Intakes of Additional Selected Vitamins and Minerals (United States)[a]

Age (years)	Vitamins		
	Biotin (µg)		Pantothenic Acid (mg)
Infants			
0–0.5	10		2
0.5–1	15		3
Children			
1–3	20		3
4–6	25		3–4
7–10	30		4–5
11 +	30–100		4–7
Adults	30–100		4–7

Age (years)	Trace Elements[b]				
	Chromium (µg)	Molybdenum (µg)	Copper (mg)	Manganese (mg)	Fluoride (mg)
Infants					
0–0.5	10–40	15–30	0.4–0.6	0.3–0.6	0.1–0.5
0.5–1	20–60	20–40	0.6–0.7	0.6–1.0	0.2–1.0
Children					
1–3	20–80	25–50	0.7–1.0	1.0–1.5	0.5–1.5
4–6	30–120	30–75	1.0–1.5	1.5–2.0	1.0–2.5
7–10	50–200	50–150	1.0–2.0	2.0–3.0	1.5–2.5
11 +	50–200	75–250	1.5–2.5	2.0–5.0	1.5–2.5
Adults	50–200	75–250	1.3–3.0	2.0–5.0	1.5–4.0

[a]Because there is less information on which to base allowances, these figures are not given in the main table of the RDA and are provided here in the form of ranges of recommended intakes.
[b]Because the toxic levels for many trace elements may be only several times usual intakes, the upper levels for the trace elements given in this table should not be habitually exceeded.

Estimated Minimum Requirements of Sodium, Chloride, and Potassium

Age (years)	Sodium[a] (mg)	Chloride (mg)	Potassium[b] (mg)
Infants			
0.0–0.5	120	180	500
0.5–1.0	200	300	700
Children			
1	225	350	1000
2–5	300	500	1400
6–9	400	600	1600
Adolescents	500	750	2000
Adults	500	750	2000

[a]Sodium requirements are based on estimates of needs for growth and for replacement of obligatory losses. They cover a wide variation of physical activity patterns and climatic exposure but do not provide for large, prolonged losses from the skin through sweat.
[b]Dietary potassium may benefit the prevention and treatment of hypertension and recommendations to include many servings of fruits and vegetables would raise potassium intakes to about 3500 mg/day.

Recommended Dietary Allowances (RDA), 1989[a]

Age (years)	Weight (kg)	Weight (lb)	Height (cm)	Height (inches)	Protein (g)	(RE) Vitamin A	(µg) Vitamin D	(mg) Vitamin E	(µg) Vitamin K	(mg) Vitamin C	(mg) Thiamin	(mg) Riboflavin	(mg equiv.) Niacin	(mg) Vitamin B$_6$	(µg) Folate	(µg) Vitamin B$_{12}$	(mg) Calcium	(mg) Phosphorus	(mg) Magnesium	(mg) Iron	(mg) Zinc	(µg) Iodine	(µg) Selenium
Infants																							
0.0–0.5	6	13	60	24	13	375	7.5	3	5	30	0.3	0.4	5	0.3	25	0.3	400	300	40	6	5	40	10
0.5–1.0	9	20	71	28	14	375	10	4	10	35	0.4	0.5	6	0.6	35	0.5	600	500	60	10	5	50	15
Children																							
1–3	13	29	90	35	16	400	10	6	15	40	0.7	0.8	9	1.0	50	0.7	800	800	80	10	10	70	20
4–6	20	44	112	44	24	500	10	7	20	45	0.9	1.1	12	1.1	75	1.0	800	800	120	10	10	90	20
7–10	28	62	132	52	28	700	10	7	30	45	1.0	1.2	13	1.4	100	1.4	800	800	170	10	10	120	30
Males																							
11–14	45	99	157	62	45	1000	10	10	45	50	1.3	1.5	17	1.7	150	2.0	1200	1200	270	12	15	150	40
15–18	66	145	176	69	59	1000	10	10	65	60	1.5	1.8	20	2.0	200	2.0	1200	1200	400	12	15	150	50
19–24	72	160	177	70	58	1000	10	10	70	60	1.5	1.7	19	2.0	200	2.0	1200	1200	350	10	15	150	70
25–50	79	174	176	70	63	1000	5	10	80	60	1.5	1.7	19	2.0	200	2.0	800	800	350	10	15	150	70
51+	77	170	173	68	63	1000	5	10	80	60	1.2	1.4	15	2.0	200	2.0	800	800	350	10	15	150	70
Females																							
11–14	46	101	157	62	46	800	10	8	45	50	1.1	1.3	15	1.4	150	2.0	1200	1200	280	15	12	150	45
15–18	55	120	163	64	44	800	10	8	55	60	1.1	1.3	15	1.5	180	2.0	1200	1200	300	15	12	150	50
19–24	58	128	164	65	46	800	10	8	60	60	1.1	1.3	15	1.6	180	2.0	1200	1200	280	15	12	150	55
25–50	63	138	163	64	50	800	5	8	65	60	1.1	1.3	15	1.6	180	2.0	800	800	280	15	12	150	55
51+	65	143	160	63	50	800	5	8	65	60	1.0	1.2	13	1.6	180	2.0	800	800	280	10	12	150	55
Pregnant					60	800	10	10	65	70	1.5	1.6	17	2.2	400	2.2	1200	1200	320	30	15	175	65
Lactating																							
1st 6 mo					65	1300	10	12	65	95	1.6	1.8	20	2.1	280	2.6	1200	1200	355	15	19	200	75
2nd 6 mo					62	1200	10	11	65	90	1.6	1.7	20	2.1	260	2.6	1200	1200	340	15	16	200	75

[a]The allowances are intended to provide for individual variations among most normal, healthy people in the United States under usual environmental stresses. Diets should be based on a variety of common foods in order to provide other nutrients for which human requirements have been less well defined. See the text for a more detailed discussion of the RDA and of nutrients not tabulated.

Fat-Soluble Vitamins

Vitamins are organic compounds (compounds that contain carbon), and of the 13 that your body needs, four are called fat-soluble (A, D, E, and K). Fat-soluble vitamins do not dissolve in water and are stored in your body's fat. As a result, these vitamins can build up in the tissues and become quite toxic (specifically vitamins A and D).

Vitamin A (Retinol)

Like Mom always said, eat plenty of carrots and you'll see in the dark. That's because carrots contain beta-carotene, a substance that is converted into vitamin A by your body. Vitamin A promotes good vision, as well as healthy skin and the normal growth and maintenance of your bones, teeth, and mucus membranes. What Mom didn't tell you was that beta-carotene is also found in most orange-yellow fruits and vegetables, along with dark-green vegetables.

Your body converts beta-carotene into vitamin A only when you need it, so eating foods rich in beta-carotene cannot cause vitamin A toxicity. However, eating huge amounts may turn your skin slightly orange. Not to worry, this condition isn't serious. Simply lay off the orange veggies for a few days and the color will disappear.

While your body controls the creation of vitamin A from beta-carotene, it has no control when you ingest straight vitamin A, which can be found in vitamin tablets. Over-supplementation can be extremely toxic, resulting in general fatigue and weakness, severe headaches, blurred vision, insomnia, hair loss, menstrual irregularities, skin rashes, and joint pain. In extreme cases there can be liver and brain damage. If huge doses are taken in the pre-natal period, it can cause birth defects.

What happens if you don't get enough? Vitamin A deficiency can cause night blindness, total blindness, and lowered resistance to infection, because vitamin A plays a key role in the structural integrity of your cells. Here come the germs!

Foods rich in vitamin A:	Foods rich in beta-carotene:
liver	cantaloupe
eggs	carrots
milk	sweet potato
butter	winter squash
margarine	spinach
	broccoli

Vitamin D: The Sunshine Vitamin

Can you believe that this vitamin can be made from the sun? I guess it's just another reason to move to Florida (first Disney World, now this). Vitamin D plays an indispensable role in building and maintaining strong bones and teeth. In fact, vitamin D is responsible for the body's absorption and utilization of the mineral calcium.

Insufficient amounts of vitamin D can lead to serious bone abnormalities, including rickets in children (bones that are soft and malformed), and osteoporosis or osteomalacia (softening of the bone) in adults.

On the other hand, vitamin D is fat-soluble, so taking large supplemental doses can become very dangerous. Some of the toxic effects involve drowsiness, diarrhea, loss of appetite, headaches, high blood pressure, high cholesterol, fragile bones, and calcium deposits throughout your body (including your heart, kidneys, and blood vessels). If you are taking supplements, make sure you are not getting more than the RDA (400 IU) of vitamin D on a daily basis.

Foods rich in vitamin D include:

fortified milk	margarine
egg yolk	tuna
exposure to sun	salmon
	cod-liver oil

A form of cholesterol in your skin is converted into vitamin D after you are exposed to sunlight for 10–20 minutes. What's more, three sunny days per week provides you with all the vitamin D you need.

Vitamin E (Tocopherols)

Talk about a hottopic! Everyone from scientists to milkmen seem to think this vitamin has tremendous abilities. I'm waiting to hear that vitamin E can pay your past due parking tickets, or jump-start your car! In a later section I'll explain vitamin E's role as an antioxidant, but for now, let's investigate it's traditional side.

Vitamin E aids the formation and functioning of your red blood cells, muscle, and other tissues, and protects essential fatty acids (special fats that are needed by your body). Because vitamin E is found in a variety of foods, deficiency is rare. However, an extreme case of vitamin E deficiency involves wasting of the muscles and neurological disorders. To date, there have been no shown toxic effects from taking doses well over the RDA.

Foods rich in vitamin E include:

vegetable oils	margarine
salad dressings	whole-grain cereals
green leafy vegetables	nuts and seeds
peanut butter	wheat germ

Vitamin K

Thanks to vitamin K, you won't bleed to death after an injury. That's because vitamin K is essential for normal blood clotting. Current research also suggests that this vitamin may play a role in maintaining strong bones in the elderly. Where do you get this vitamin? Interestingly enough, bacteria that live in your intestines help to make 80% of the vitamin K that you need, and the rest can be found in a variety of foods listed below.

A vitamin K deficiency can cause hemorrhaging (uncontrollable bleeding), mainly seen in newborn infants since their immature intestinal tracts may not have enough bacteria to make this vitamin. In addition, people taking antibiotics may temporarily lose the ability to make vitamin K because the medication destroys all bacteria, good and bad.

Foods rich in vitamin K include:

dark-green leafy vegetables

liver

Water-Soluble Vitamins

Unlike fat-soluble vitamins, water-soluble vitamins can easily dissolve in the watery fluids of your body. Because excessive amounts are generally excreted in the urine, there is less chance for toxic side effects, but more chance for deficiencies. Therefore, it is important to regularly replenish these vitamins by eating healthy foods that supply ample amounts. Be extra careful during food preparation. Since some of these vitamins are easily washed away or destroyed by light, air, and heat, use small amounts of water, avoid overcooking, and only cut your fruits and vegetables right before you eat them. The following provides a quick rundown on each of the nine water-soluble vitamins, eight B-vitamins, and vitamin C.

Q and A

Why are vitamins classified as B-1, B-2, B-3, only to skip to B-6 then B-12? What about all the numbers in between?

At various points in time, substances were in fact labeled B-7, B-8, B-9, and so on. However, with further investigation, scientists found out that these were either duplicates of already known vitamins, or not vitamins after all. As a result, those numbers were wiped off the list.

Thiamin (B-1)

Thiamin is needed for the conversion of carbohydrate-rich foods into energy. B-1 also plays a role in keeping your brain, nerve, and heart cells healthy. A deficiency will lead to loss of energy, nausea, depression, muscle cramps, nerve damage, and muscular weakness. Although uncommon in the United States, a severe depletion of thiamin can result in the disease beriberi, causing potential muscle wasting and paralysis.

Foods rich in thiamin (B-6) include:		
pork	lamb	beef
liver	whole-grain products	peas
seeds	legumes	

Rocky Road

Watch out for "stress tabs" with extra B-vitamins. Your body will only recognize and absorb a certain amount of each B-vitamin, the rest gets sent down the drain. If you seem to be less stressed after popping one of the pills, chances are it's psychological!

Riboflavin (B-2)

Like its buddy thiamin, riboflavin plays a key role in the metabolism of energy. Furthermore, this vitamin is involved in the formation of red blood cells and is necessary for healthy skin and normal vision.

A riboflavin deficiency will cause dry, scaly skin, accompanied by cracks on your lips and in the corners of your mouth. And if that's not enough, getting insufficient amounts can also make your eyes extremely sensitive to the light.

Foods rich in riboflavin (B-2) include:	
milk	yogurt
cheese	whole-grain breads and cereals
green leafy vegetables	meat food products fortified with B-vitamins

Note: This vitamin is easily destroyed with exposure to sunlight, therefore store these foods in the fridge, cabinet, or pantry.

Niacin (B-3)

This B-vitamin is also involved in energy-producing reactions in the cells that convert food to energy. In addition, niacin helps maintain healthy skin, nerves, and your digestive system. In some instances, large doses of niacin can be used as a cholesterol lowering medication. However, this should only be done under the supervision of your doctor. Megadoses can cause hot flashes, itching, ulcers, high blood sugar, and liver damage.

In the rare case of a niacin deficiency, symptoms include diarrhea, mouth sores, changes in the skin, nervous disorders, and pellagra disease known to cause the "Four Ds": diarrhea, dermatitis, dementia (mental confusion), and death.

Foods rich in niacin (B-3) include:		
meat	fish	poultry
liver	milk	eggs
nuts	whole-grains	enriched breads and cereals

Pyridoxine (B-6)

Vitamin B-6 is a vital component for chemical reactions involving proteins and amino acids (remember those protein building blocks?). It also participates in the formation of red blood cells, antibodies, and insulin, in addition to maintaining normal brain function. Deficiency causes skin changes, convulsions in infants, dementia, nervous disorders, and anemia.

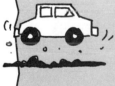

Rocky Road

Beware of supplements claiming to relieve "premenstrual syndrome." They usually contain large amounts of B-6 (doses of 100mg or more taken over a consistent period of time) that can lead to serious neurological damage, such as loss of feeling in fingers and legs. By the way, they don't help relieve PMS.

Foods rich in pyridoxine (B-6) include:		
lean meats	poultry	fish
legumes	green leafy vegetables	whole-grain cereals
bananas		

Cobalamin (B-12)

This vitamin assists in the formation of red blood cells, the normal functioning of your nervous system, and is required for the synthesis of DNA (your genetic resume). Since B-12 is only found in foods of animal origin, strict vegetarians may need to take a supplement in order to avoid a deficiency. Furthermore, this unique vitamin needs the help of another substance called *intrinsic factor* to be absorbed. Since intrinsic factor is made by the lining of the stomach, people with gastrointestinal disorders (especially in the elderly) may need to get B-12 shots directly into the bloodstream. Symptoms of B-12 deficiency include nervous disorders and pernicious anemia.

Because a good amount of vitamin B-12 can be stored in the liver, it may take years for a deficiency to be recognized. As a result, people should have their B-12 levels checked starting at age 60, and every decade thereafter.

Foods rich in cobalamin (B-12) include:	
meat	fish
poultry	eggs
milk products	

Folic Acid (Folacin, Folate)

Folic acid appropriately gets its name from the word *foliage* since it's primarily found in leafy, dark-green vegetables. In addition to playing a vital role in cell division and red blood cell formation, this vitamin is needed to make the genetic material DNA.

In recent years, folic acid has gained a lot of attention for its ability to reduce neural tube birth defects in newborn babies. Needless to say, it is imperative that pregnant mothers and women of childbearing years (since some women do not even know they are pregnant until after the fact), get appropriate amounts of folic acid by both foods and/or supplementation. For this reason, folic acid is a key ingredient in most prenatal vitamins. Because this nutrient is involved in cell division, a deficiency will leave you vulnerable to anemia and an abnormal digestive function since your blood cells and cells of the intestinal tract divide most rapidly.

Foods rich in folic acid include:	
leafy green vegetables	liver
beans	peas

Pantothenic Acid and Biotin

Pantothenic acid and biotin are both part of the "B-vitamin gang" that participates in the metabolism of energy. In addition, pantothenic acid also plays a role in the formation of certain hormones and neurotransmitters. Although both vitamins are vital for normal functioning, as of today there isn't a set RDA for either one. This is because deficiencies are so rare, and they are both found in a wide variety of plant and animal foods.

Vitamin C (Ascorbic Acid)

Now for the million dollar question, "Can vitamin C ward off the common cold?" The scientists say no! To date, there is no documented evidence supporting this notion. Interestingly enough, this vitamin may lessen the severity of those lousy symptoms experienced *during* a cold because vitamin C has a mild antihistaminic effect.

What else can vitamin C do? Let's just say if all the vitamins and minerals were on a pay-scale according to the jobs they perform, vitamin C would be Rockefeller! Vitamin C wears many hats, from helping to keep your bones, teeth, and blood vessels healthy, to healing wounds, boosting your resistance to infection, and participating in the formation of collagen (a protein that helps support body structures). Another benefit from eating vitamin C-rich foods is that you increase the absorption of the mineral iron, good news for people with greater iron requirements or deficiencies.

Definition
Scurvy: A disease resulting from a deficiency of vitamin C, characterized by bleeding and swollen gums, joint pain, muscle wasting, and bruises. Scurvy is now rare, except among alcoholics, and can be cured by as little as five to seven milligrams of vitamin C.

Rocky Road
For reasons that are unclear, cigarette smokers seem to require 50% more of vitamin C than non-smokers. Instead of popping more vitamin C, why not just quit smoking?

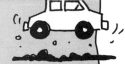

Although vitamin C deficiency is uncommon, it can cause a lowered resistance to infection, sore gums, hemorrhages, and in severe cases, the disease scurvy.

On the flipside, some studies have shown that megadosing on vitamin C may help reduce the risk of certain diseases (this will be further discussed in the section on antioxidants). However, large doses may also lead to uncomfortable side effects, including diarrhea and nausea. For this reason, it is savvy to obtain extra amounts through food sources, not supplements.

Foods rich in vitamin C include:

citrus fruits (oranges, grapefruits, etc.)	melons
berries	tomatoes
potatoes	broccoli
fortified juices	

Vitamins fall into two classes: fat-soluble and water-soluble.

Fat-soluble vitamins	Water-soluble vitamins
vitamin A	B vitamins
vitamin D	thiamin
vitamin E	riboflavin
vitamin K	niacin
	vitamin B-6
	folate
	vitamin B-12
	pantothenic acid
	biotin
	vitamin C

A Day in the Life of an Antioxidant

Rocky Road

Although beta-carotene is still considered a powerful antioxidant, it is no longer recommended in supplemental form. Several recently published studies found that smokers who took beta-carotene supplements showed an increased risk of lung cancer. However, these findings certainly do not mean that beta-carotene has lost any importance among the antioxidant world. It *does* mean that until we have further information, people should solely focus on getting beta-carotene from food sources rather than supplemental megadoses.

Definition
Free radicals can be described as unstable, hyper-active atoms that literally trek around your body damaging healthy cells and tissue.

It's the hottest news around town: antioxidants reduce your risk for heart disease and certain cancers. So what exactly are antioxidants and how do they work?

As you know, every cell in your body needs oxygen to function normally. Unfortunately, the utilization of this oxygen produces harmful by-products called *free radicals*. What's more, free radicals are also created from environmental pollution, certain industrial chemicals, and smoking.

Outside the body, the process of oxidation is responsible for a sliced apple turning brown (you know, the apple nobody will eat) and the rusting of metal. Inside the body, oxidation contributes to heart disease, cancer, cataracts, aging, and a slew of other degenerative diseases. So in other words, free radicals are the enemy!

So why isn't everyone falling apart? Your cells have their own special defense technique to fight off these radical monsters. What's more, scientists have unfolded compelling evidence suggesting that certain vitamins (specifically C, E, and beta-carotene) can actually enhance your body's ability to ward off these free radicals and therefore prevent oxidation. Appropriately we call these vitamins antioxidants.

What Can Antioxidants Do?

To date, numerous studies have shown that antioxidants may protect against the following:

➤ **Cardiovascular disease.** Findings from studies suggest that vitamins C and E may play a role in future strategies for heart disease prevention by reducing the amount of LDL-cholesterol lodged in the arteries (remember these bad guys from an earlier chapter?).

➤ **Cancer.** Studies suggest that vitamins E, C, and beta-carotene may have a protective effect against several types of cancers. Keep in mind that many factors appear to influence the development of cancer, including heredity, smoking, nutritional excesses/deficiencies, and the environment.

➤ **Cataracts.** Scientists suspect that cataracts develop from the oxidation of the proteins in the lens of the eye. Antioxidants may help to reduce the risk of developing this disease.

➤ **Immunity.** Researchers theorize that antioxidants may help to strengthen the immune system by preventing the action of free radicals.

➤ **Exercise-induced free radical damage.** Recent studies have shown increased free radical activity following strenuous exercise. Therefore, vitamin E may play a role in reducing muscle inflammation and soreness after bouts of vigorous workouts.

How Much Antioxidants Is Appropriate?

Your primary (and secondary) focus should be on eating *foods* rich in antioxidant vitamins. Contrary to what people may think, there are no magic bullets (or pills) to good health. Wouldn't life be so much easier! Another plug for food is that scientists are constantly discovering new food substances that may help with the quest for well-being. Furthermore, future findings may even reveal that it's not just one isolated vitamin, but interactions between several food ingredients that enhance disease prevention.

Food for Thought
Popeye was sure on to something. With just one can of spinach (2 cups), he swallowed down about 29,000 international units of beta-carotene, 50 milligrams of vitamin C, and 12 milligrams of vitamin E. That's one heck of a healthy sailor!

To date, no harmful side effects have been reported from supplemental doses well above the RDA for vitamins E and C, but who knows what will be revealed in the future. The science of nutrition is constantly being challenged with new discoveries—something to think about before popping the next pill. We know that getting your nutrients from food sources is safe and effective, but we don't know everything about supplemental megadosing. Take beta-carotene for example. Last year, this nutrient was the "cure all," and everyone was popping the stuff. Today this picture has changed substantially.

The bottom line: If you decide to take antioxidant supplements, stay on top of the current research and speak with a competent health professional.

The Scoop on Minerals

Here is a brief introduction to the world of minerals. The following chapter will focus on two powerhouse minerals: calcuim and iron.

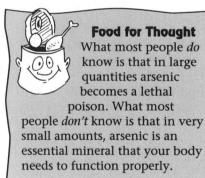

Food for Thought
What most people *do* know is that in large quantities arsenic becomes a lethal poison. What most people *don't* know is that in very small amounts, arsenic is an essential mineral that your body needs to function properly.

Together with vitamins, at least 22 minerals are needed by your body to make things happen. Major-minerals such as calcium and potassium are needed in large amounts, while trace-minerals like iron and zinc are only required in minute amounts.

But don't be fooled, just because a mineral is classified as trace, doesn't mean it is any less important. The small RDA for iron is just as important to your body as the large RDA for calcium. Sort of like bread; lots of flour with a drop of yeast...both equally important for that perfect baked loaf.

Major-minerals	Trace-minerals
Calcium	Iron
Chloride	Zinc
Magnesium	Iodine
Phosphorus	Selenium
Potassium	Copper
Sodium	Manganese

Major-minerals	Trace-minerals
Sulfur	Fluoride
	Chromium
	Molybdenum
	Arsenic
	Nickel
	Silicon
	Boron
	Cobalt

The Least You Need to Know

➤ More than 13 vitamins and 22 minerals are essential for normal body function. Eating a well-balanced, varied diet will supply your body with the Recommended Dietary Allowances for all nutrients.

➤ Water-soluble vitamins (eight B-complex vitamins and vitamin C) can easily dissolve in the watery body fluids and excessive amounts are generally excreted through the urine.

➤ Fat-soluble vitamins, (A, D, E, and K) do not dissolve in water and are stored in the body's fat. As a result, these vitamins have the potential to build up in tissues and become quite toxic with large supplemental doses (specifically A and D).

➤ Antioxidants may help to prevent certain cancers, heart disease, cataracts, exercise-induced soreness, and other degenerative diseases by protecting against free radical damage. Eat plenty of foods rich in vitamins C and E to reap the benefits!

Chapter 8

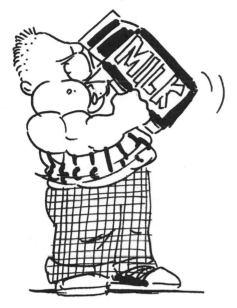

Two Powerhouse Minerals: Calcium and Iron

As you've learned from the previous chapter, there are at least 22 minerals that are essential for a number of vital functions and body processes. It seems as if not a single day goes by without either a client or friend asking for some sort of information regarding calcium or iron. Because of this, I've singled out these two impressive minerals and dedicated an entire chapter to the various questions regarding the two powerhouse minerals.

Calcium and Healthy Bones

Calcium is by far the most abundant mineral in your body with about 99 percent of the stuff stored in your bones. The other 1 percent is located in your body fluids, where it helps to regulate functions such as blood pressure, nerve transmission, muscle contraction (including the heart beat), clotting of blood, and the secretion of hormones and digestive enzymes. Make no bones about it, calcium, along with the help of vitamin D, fluoride, and phosphorus, is best known for its ability to promote strong, healthy bones. Calcium serves a vital role as part of bone structure, providing integrity and density to your skeleton. In turn, your bones act as a "calcium bank," releasing calcium into your body when your diet may be deficient (hopefully not too often).

Many people believe that once you are past a certain age, you do not have to worry about getting enough calcium. WRONG! Adequate calcium is important *throughout* your life; first and foremost, for optimal bone building, and later on for bone maintenance. Generally, the first 24 years are important because your body is laying down the foundation for strong skeletal bones and teeth. In the first three decades of life, your bones reach their *peak adult bone mass* (bones are done growing in size and density). Children who drink plenty of milk and eat other dairy products will enter adulthood with stronger bones than those who skimp on calcium-rich foods.

Calcium intake in the later years is equally important for maintaining healthy bones (hopefully you have already done all the right things in your first 30 years). With age, your bones gradually lose their density (i.e., calcium), which is especially true in menopausal women. People that regularly take in adequate amounts of calcium can help slow down this process and defy those brittle bones of old age.

Q and A

Why bother with calcium?

Imagine your bones as your calcium bank. Over the years you can develop quite an extensive savings account by taking in plenty of calcium-rich foods and supplementing your diet with calcium pills. Keep up the good work as an adult and your bones stay calcium-rich!

On the other hand, regularly skimp on this mineral and you'll wind up calcium broke! Your body fluids still need calcium to regulate normal body functions. What these fluids don't get from food must be borrowed from the calcium-bone bank. Borrowing day after day, year after year, will deplete the savings account and leave you with osteoporosis (brittle bones that break easily).

Q and A

Should I take calcium supplements?

If you are having a problem consistently getting enough calcium from food sources, you may want to speak with your doctor about supplementation. Stick with a calcium supplement in the form of **calcium carbonate** or **calcium citrate** and do not take more 500 milligrams in one dose (anything more than 500 mg will not be absorbed). Also be aware that most calcium supplements need to be taken with food or juice for proper absorption.

How Much Calcium Is Recommended?

The RDA for calcium is 1,200 milligrams for children, teenagers, young adults (up to 24 years), and pregnant and lactating women. The RDA for most other populations is 800 milligrams. Despite the listed RDAs, leading calcium experts suggest that most populations can benefit from even higher daily intakes, as shown below:

Optimal Calcium Requirements

Group	Optimal Daily Intake (mg)
Infants	
Birth–6 months	400
6 months–1 year	600
Children	
1–5 years	800
6–10 years	800–1,200
Adolescents/Young Adults	
11–24 years	1,200–1,500
Men	
25–65 years	1,000
Over 65 years	1,500
Women	
25–50 years	1,000
Over 50 years (post-menopausal)	
On estrogen	1,000
Not on estrogen	1,500
Over 65 years	1,500
Pregnant and nursing	1,200–1,500

Source: Optimal Calcium Intake.
NIH Consensus Statement 1994 Jun 6-8; 12(4): 1-31.

Are You Getting Enough Calcium? The Foods to Choose From

Browse through the chart below and notice that dairy foods, along with fortified juice and sardines, provide the most calcium hands down. One more thing: Don't be put off by the high amounts of fat in cheese. Simply shop for the low-fat brands in your local store. They have less fat, but still retain ample amounts of calcium.

The Best Sources of Calcium in Various Foods

Milk Group	Amount	Calcium in mg
Yogurt, plain (low-fat)	1 cup	415
Yogurt, fruit-flavored (low-fat)	1 cup	345
Milk, nonfat (dry)	1/4 cup	377
Milk, skim	1 cup	302
Milk, 1%-2%	1 cup	300
Milk, whole*	1 cup	291
Buttermilk	1 cup	285
Milk, chocolate (low-fat)	1 cup	284
Cheese, parmesan (grated)	1/4 cup	338
Cheese, Swiss*	1 oz.	272
Cheese, monterey jack*	1 oz.	212
Cheese, mozzarella low moisture, part skim	1 oz.	207
Cheese, cheddar*	1 oz.	204
Cheese, colby*	1 oz.	194
Cheese, American*	1 oz.	174
Ice cream*	1/2 cup	88
Cottage cheese, creamed 1%	1/2 cup	63
Fruit and Vegetable Group	Amount	Calcium in mg
Collards, cooked	1/2 cup	168
Turnip greens, cooked	1/2 cup	134
Kale, cooked	1/2 cup	103
Spinach, cooked	1/2 cup	84
Broccoli, cooked	1/2 cup	68

Fruit and Vegetable Group	Amount	Calcium in mg
Chard, cooked	¹/₂ cup	64
Carrot, raw	1 med.	27
Orange	1 med.	60
Dates, chopped	¹/₄ cup	26
Raisins	¹/₄ cup	22

Protein Group (meat, beans, eggs)	Amount	Calcium in mg
Sardines (canned, w/bones)	3 oz.	372
Salmon, pink (canned, w/bones)	3 oz.	165
Tofu (processed, w/calcium)	4 oz.	145
Almonds, shelled*	1 oz.	66
Soybeans, cooked	¹/₂ cup	66
Dried beans, cooked (lima, navy, kidney)	¹/₂ cup	35-48
Egg	1 large	27
Peanut Butter*	2 Tbsp.	18
Beef patty, cooked (21% fat)*	3 oz.	9

Grain Group	Amount	Calcium in mg
Calcium fortified cereals (Total) w/milk	1 oz. with ¹/₂ cup milk	350
Farina, enriched (instant, cooked)	1 cup	189
Tortilla, corn	1 medium	60
Bread, whole wheat	1 slice	25

Calcium-Fortified Foods	Amount	Calcium in mg
Orange juice and grapefruit juice (Citrus Hill, Minute Maid)	8 oz.	300
Calcium fortified cereals (Total)	1 cup	300

Denotes foods that are also high in fat.
Source: Calcium Information Center

Iron Out Your Body

Iron deficiency is the most widespread type of vitamin or mineral deficiency in the world. Do you constantly experience sluggishness, irritability, and headaches? Perhaps you suffer from this condition. Let's take a closer look and find out.

About 70 percent of the iron in your body is located in a portion of your red blood cells known as hemoglobin. Hemoglobin is your oxygen delivery service, supplying every cell with the oxygen it needs to perform essential metabolic functions. Iron is also a component of myoglobin. Like the hemoglobin in red blood cells, myoglobin ensures adequate oxygen delivery to all your muscles. At this point, I'm sure you are starting to understand the importance of iron in this equation—too little iron, too little oxygen. The end result is fatigue, irritability, weakness, headaches, tendency to feel cold, and in the case of severe depletion, iron-deficiency anemia.

Fortunately, iron is found in a variety of animal and plant foods, making it easy to get your daily requirement. *Heme* iron, the type found in animal products (red meats, liver, fish, poultry, and eggs), is more readily absorbed than *nonheme* iron, which can be found in vegetables and other plant foods (beans, nuts, seeds, dried fruits, and fortified breads and cereals). Interestingly enough, the body adjusts the amount it absorbs according to the body's need. In other words, a person with iron-deficient anemia will absorb about two to three times more iron after eating exactly the same meal than a person with normal iron status.

Certain groups of people are at increased risk for developing an iron deficiency. If you think you may fall into one of the following categories, ask your doctor to check your iron status before self-prescribing supplementation (a simple blood test can tell if you are deficient).

Groups at risk for iron deficiency:

➤ Infants and children. Their rapid growth and finicky eating habits demand that they get iron in a variety of ways.

➤ Women who bleed heavily during menstruation. They lose iron-rich blood each month.

➤ Pregnant women. They are supporting their growing baby's needs as well as their own.

➤ Strict vegetarians who take in only nonheme sources of iron. Remember, nonheme plant foods are *much* less absorbent than iron-rich animal foods.

➤ People who lose a lot of blood during surgery or other bleeding injuries.

➤ "Chronic dieters" who bounce from one crash diet to another. People suffering from eating disorders who may not eat enough iron-rich foods to meet their requirements.

Tips to Boost Your Dietary Iron Intake

➤ Make a point of eating iron-rich foods, both animal (heme) and non-animal (nonheme) sources each day.

➤ When eating nonheme foods, couple with some vitamin C (see the list of vitamin C containing foods). Vitamin C can increase the absorption of iron.

➤ Avoid drinking coffee or tea with a iron-rich meal, they inhibit the absorption of iron.

➤ Calcium interferes with the absorption of iron, so if you take calcium supplements do not take them with an iron-rich meal. Try them with a snack or some juice since you usually do need some food for your calcium pills.

➤ Cook casseroles, stews, and sauces in cast iron cookware. Believe it or not, some of the iron will seep into the food.

➤ The presence of heme-iron (even very small amounts) at a meal with nonheme iron will enhance the absorption of the nonheme iron.

Heme and Nonheme Foods

Best Sources of Iron (Heme):

lean red meats	turkey
chicken	fish and seafood
pork	lamb
veal	eggs
liver (although very high in cholesterol)	

Good Iron Sources (Nonheme):

beans	lentils
iron-fortified cereals and other grains	dried fruit
broccoli	spinach
collard greens	nuts
blackstrap molasses	seeds

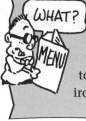

Definition

Iron Toxicity: Although not very common, iron toxicity is a serious problem that occurs from either a genetic abnormality causing the body to store excessive amounts, or the unnecessary over-supplementation of iron. The result can be liver and other organ damage.

Are You a Candidate for a Vitamin/Mineral Supplement?

This is the time to ask yourself, "Will I benefit from a nutritional supplement?" Ideally, you should be getting your daily supply of vitamins and minerals from your diet, not from pill-popping. While there are exceptions to this rule, don't abandon good eating habits for a little brown bottle—it just doesn't work that way. Generally speaking, nutrients from food are absorbed more readily by your body, the way nature intended. Furthermore, food provides you with energy in the form of calories—something you don't get from pills. Imagine an overweight man holding a candy bar in one hand, and a crumbled McDonald's bag in the other hand. "Not to worry," he says, "I took a vitamin this morning!" That's a joke, but who is he kidding?

While pill-popping is not the most desired method of getting your nutrients, some people do need assistance to receive the required daily allowances. Check out the following list to see if you fall into one of the categories that require a little help. If you do, speak with your doctor or a registered dietitian (a registered dietitian, or R.D., is a nutritionist with the proper education and credentials) about appropriate supplementation.

Groups at nutritional risk:

➤ Do you constantly skip meals, grabbing only snack foods throughout the day? Do you eat fewer than five fruits and vegetables each day? You may benefit from a multi-vitamin/mineral supplement (supplying up to 100% of the RDAs) to fill in the nutrition gaps.

➤ Are you a vegan (strict vegetarian who consumes absolutely no meat, dairy, or other animal products)? You may benefit from a supplement that supplies the RDA for vitamins D and B-12 and the mineral calcium.

➤ Are you over 60 years old? People in this category may have a decline in the absorption of the following vitamins: B-6, B-12, C, D, E, folic acid, and the mineral calcium. A one-a-day multi-vitamin/mineral may provide some extra backup.

➤ Do you regularly drink alcohol or smoke? Excessive amounts of alcohol and smoking interfere with the body's ability to absorb and utilize certain vitamins and minerals. In this case, a supplement recommendation is not the advice. I think you get the picture!

➤ Are you on/off every wacky fad diet out there? (You'd better not say yes after reading Chapter 22.) Chances are you're cheating your body of important nutrients and would probably benefit from the backup of a one-a-day multi-vitamin/mineral supplement.

➤ Do you completely avoid specific types of foods? Some people stay away from certain foods for reasons including food allergies, intolerances, or just plain dislike. In these cases, supplements of specific nutrients may be needed.

For women only:

➤ Do you experience heavy bleeding during monthly menstruation? If so, you may lose iron-rich blood. Check with your doctor and see if you will benefit from taking a supplement with iron.

➤ Are you currently pregnant or breast-feeding? Women in this category have greater needs for the vitamins A, C, B-1, B-6, B-12, and folic acid, as well as the minerals iron and calcium. These extra amounts are usually included in prenatal vitamins.

The Least You Need to Know

➤ Adequate calcium intake is required throughout the lifecycle; the early years for bone building, and the later years for bone maintenance. Make it a habit to load up on low-fat dairy products and other calcium-rich foods.

➤ The mineral iron is responsible for delivering oxygen to every cell in your body and is found in a variety of foods.

➤ *Heme* iron, the most absorbable type, is found in animal products such as meat, liver, poultry, seafood, and eggs. *Nonheme* iron, found in plants, is less absorbable and is found in dried fruits, nuts, beans, seeds, and fortified grains.

➤ Boost the absorption rate of iron by combining foods high in vitamin C with an iron-rich meal (i.e., iron-fortified cereal with a glass of orange juice).

➤ While certain groups of people can benefit from vitamin/mineral supplementation, most nutrition experts agree that a well-balanced diet should be your primary focus for optimal nutrition.

➤ If you think you may be a candidate for supplementation, speak with your doctor or a nutritionist who is a registered dietitian.

Part 2
Making Savvy Food Choices

Decisions, decisions! With all the gazillions of foods offered in grocery stores, restaurants, delis, and even your own kitchen, it's a nightmare trying to decide what to eat—let alone something nutritious to eat. But it shouldn't be that way. In fact, thanks to the growing number of health-conscience consumers, most grocery stores and restaurants are now well-equipped to cater to your special food concerns. You simply need to know what to look for.

This part covers every angle. You'll learn how to decode the information on nutrition labels so you can make better-informed food choices in your local grocery store. Then, we'll put your know-how into action by scouting out the supermarket, aisle by aisle, introducing you to the smart food items to load into your shopping cart. You'll also master low-fat cooking techniques so you're ready to wow your friends, family, and taste buds with some knockout meals at home. And you certainly won't need to give up dining out. This section will fill you in on the best bets for most all ethnic cuisine! BON APPÉTIT!

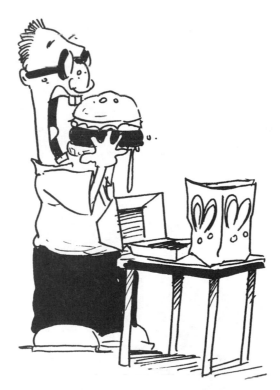

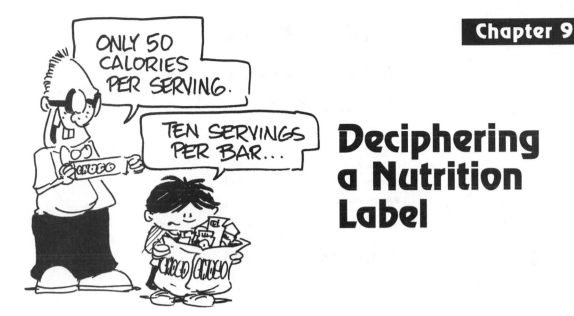

Chapter 9

Deciphering a Nutrition Label

In This Chapter

➤ How to read a nutrition label

➤ Understanding the Daily Percent Values

➤ Testing your label savvy

Now that you have some solid nutrition know-how, let's put this knowledge to work and decode all that mumbo-jumbo written on prepackaged food products. With the ability to interpret the information provided on nutrition labels, you can become quite a food detective in your local grocery store, further enhancing your skills as a healthy eater. First, it will allow you to make better informed food choices. At the same time, it will enable you to compare similar food products to see which brand is nutritionally superior. The best news of all is that the government has set up strict food label laws and regulations to prevent companies from printing misleading or falsified claims on food items, so you can actually believe what you read. Let's get to work and find out the whole truth on the foods you love to gobble down.

```
┌─────────────────────────────────────┐
│  Nutrition Facts                    │
│  Serving Size ½ cup (114g)          │
│  Servings Per Container 4           │
│ ═══════════════════════════════════ │
│  Amount Per Serving                 │
│ ─────────────────────────────────── │
│  Calories 90      Calories from Fat 30│
│ ─────────────────────────────────── │
│                      % Daily Value* │
│  Total Fat 3g                   5%  │
│ ─────────────────────────────────── │
│    Saturated Fat 0g             0%  │
│ ─────────────────────────────────── │
│  Cholesterol 0mg                0%  │
│ ─────────────────────────────────── │
│  Sodium 300mg                  13%  │
│ ─────────────────────────────────── │
│  Total Carbohydrate 13g         4%  │
│ ─────────────────────────────────── │
│    Dietary Fiber 3g            12%  │
│ ─────────────────────────────────── │
│    Sugars 3g                        │
│ ─────────────────────────────────── │
│  Protein 3g                         │
│ ═══════════════════════════════════ │
│  Vitamin A  80%   •  Vitamin C  60% │
│  Calcium     4%   •  Iron        4% │
│ ─────────────────────────────────── │
│  * Percent Daily Values are based on a 2,000│
│    calorie diet. Your daily values may be higher or│
│    lower depending on your calorie needs:│
│              Calories   2,000    2,500│
│ ─────────────────────────────────── │
│  Total Fat    Less than  65g     80g│
│   Sat Fat     Less than  20g     25g│
│  Cholesterol  Less than  300mg  300mg│
│  Sodium       Less than  2,400mg 2,400mg│
│  Total Carbohydrate      300g    375g│
│   Fiber                  25g     30g│
│ ─────────────────────────────────── │
│  Calories per gram:                 │
│  Fat 9  •  Carbohydrate 4  •  Protein 4│
└─────────────────────────────────────┘
```

Serving Size

The first order of business is to figure out how much food was analyzed by the folks who prepared the nutrition label. *Serving size* clearly describes this set amount of food. Of course, most packages contain more than one serving, and Servings Per Container refers to the total amount of single servings in the entire package. For example, the label shown above reports that a serving size is ¹/₂ cup, and there are four servings per container. Therefore there must be 2 full cups in the entire package since ¹/₂ cup × 4 = 2 cups.

Are you eating the amount of food the label defines as one serving? Remember, fat and calorie measurements on the label are for a single serving size only. And we all know, it's incredibly easy to eat more than just one measly serving. Here's a perfect example of the difference between serving size and the actual servings eaten: One serving of ice cream (¹/₂ cup) has approximately 12 grams of fat. Most of the people I know can easily eat 1 cup in a sitting, and you know what that means. When you double the serving size, you double everything, the calories, protein grams, carbohydrate grams, and, of course, the fat grams. Pay close attention to the amount of food per serving. If you choose to go over (or under) on servings, take this into consideration when reading the remaining information.

Calories

When calories are listed on a label, they refer to the amount of calories in a single serving of that food. Plain and simple. For example, take the sample label in the beginning of the chapter. It has 90 calories per serving. What about those calorie claims frequently listed on a label? Luckily, the following key words are now defined by the government and must mean what they say. Remember, these are broken down to amounts per serving.

Calorie-free: less than 5 calories per serving

Low-calorie: 40 calories or less for most foods items

                             120 calories or less for main dish products (lentil soup, turkey burger, chicken breast, etc.)

Reduced-calorie: Must be at least 25% fewer calories than the regular version of that food item.

Total Fat

This lists the total number of fat grams coming from all types of fat, saturated, monounsaturated, and polyunsaturated. As you can see, the label reveals that there are 3 grams of fat per serving. Another listing titled "Calories from Fat" converts the total fat grams into fat calories (# of fat grams × 9 = calories coming from fat). Again, the sample label reports 30 calories from fat per serving. This is a valuable piece of information since it allows you to identify the percentage of fat in a particular food. Ideally, you should try to choose foods with a big difference between the total number of calories and calories coming from fat. The bigger the gap between the two, the less the percentage of total calories coming from fat.

Here are some of the common "fat" phrases that appear on packaged food products and how they are defined by the government.

Fat-free: less than 0.5 grams of fat per serving

Low-fat: 3 grams of fat (or less) per serving

Reduced-fat: At least 25% less fat per serving than the original version of a food product

Saturated Fat

This reveals the amount of "artery clogging" fat in a food product. Even though saturated fat is part of the total fat in food, it gets a category of its own because it has the potential to be extremely bad for you. As you can see, the sample label shows no saturated fat—good deal! In general, avoid foods that are high in saturated fat. This type of fat is responsible for increasing your risk of heart disease and other illnesses.

Here are some of the common "saturated fat" phrases that appear on packaged food products and how they are defined by the government.

Saturated fat-free: less than 0.5 grams per serving

Low in saturated fat: 1 gram or less in a serving size,
                        or no more than 10% of calories
                        coming from saturated fat.

Reduced saturated fat: At least 25% less saturated
                        fat than the original version.

Cholesterol

Remember this waxy guy? Together with its partner in crime—fat—dietary cholesterol is a key player in raising blood cholesterol, and therefore increasing your risk for heart disease. You'll notice that the cholesterol content of a food product is measured in milligrams. Try to budget your foods and eat less than 300 milligrams of dietary cholesterol per day.

Understand the following claims when they appear on food labels:

Cholesterol-free: less than 2 milligrams of cholesterol
                        and 2 grams (or less) of saturated fat
                        per serving.

Low-cholesterol: 20 mg (or less) of cholesterol and 2
                        grams (or less) of saturated fat per
                        serving.

These cholesterol claims are only allowed when a food product contains 2 grams (or less) of saturated fat as well.

Sodium

Don't let the terminology confuse you. The label calls it sodium (300 mg reported on the sample label), but most people know it as salt. Remember, sodium is only a component of salt. However, that one component is responsible for water retention and high blood pressure in salt-sensitive people. Try to limit the amount of high-sodium foods in your diet and aim for a daily intake of 2,400 milligrams or less.

Here's some sodium lingo and what it means:

Sodium-free: less than 5 milligrams of sodium per serving.

Low-sodium: 140 milligrams (or less) of sodium per serving.

Reduced sodium: At least 25% less sodium than the original food version.

Total Carbohydrate

In Chapter 2 you became well versed on the various types of carbohydrates. Now you can utilize the label information to identify whether a food contains a lot of simple sugar or complex carbohydrate.

First, look for the listing titled "Total Carbohydrate." This will reveal the amount of *all types* of carbos (simple and complex) in a single serving of a food. Next, look for the smaller listing located underneath total carbohydrate titled "Sugars." This indicates how much simple sugar is in a serving of that particular food. Obviously, the less simple sugar the better. Now you're ready to determine the amount of complex carbohydrate in a food by simply subtracting the total carbs from the sugars.

Let's look at the previous label for an example:

Total Carbohydrate   13 grams

Sugars   3 grams

These numbers indicate that the majority of carbohydrates are coming from more complex sources, 10 grams to be exact.

Dietary Fiber

Another category located underneath Total Carbohydrates is Dietary Fiber. Dietary fiber is predominantly found in carbohydrate-rich foods and includes both soluble and insoluble fiber sources. Because fiber promotes regularity, along with reducing the risk of heart disease and certain cancers, try to choose foods with at least 3 grams of dietary fiber per serving, and aim for a total intake of 20–35 grams each day.

Protein

As you know from the chapter on protein, most Americans eat far more protein than they actually need (0.36 grams per pound of body weight). While some of the best protein sources, unfortunately, do not carry a nutrition label (beef, poultry, eggs, fish), nutrifacts posters are required in meat and produce departments, so take a look and ask your grocer.

On the other hand, most dairy products and prepackaged food items do list the grams of protein in a single serving. It's interesting to see that there are even small amounts of protein in foods you may not expect.

Percent Daily Values

And now for the confusing part: What are those "%" signs floating all over the label?

They are called Percent Daily Values (DV), and are based on a 2,000 calorie reference diet. In other words, these percentages indicate how much of a day's recommended amount for each nutrient is present in a single serving of a particular food (based on a 2,000 calorie diet). Of course, your job is to ultimately eat a variety of foods that supply 100% of all nutrients needed. For example: One serving of yogurt provides 35% daily calcium and 0% iron. Clearly a great source of calcium, but lousy for iron.

What happens if you eat more or less than 2,000 calories? You can slightly adjust the percentages up or down if your good with numbers (and extremely motivated). In general, the 2,000 calorie reference diet provides appropriate guidelines for almost everyone (adults and children over 4) to follow.

For total fat, saturated fat, cholesterol, and sodium try to choose foods with low percentage daily values. On the other hand, you want to choose foods with higher percent DVs for total carbohydrate, dietary fiber, and all vitamins and minerals.

The following are the set "Daily Values." They are specifically used for food labels and are based on a 2,000 calorie reference diet.

Daily Values for Nutritional Items

Food Component	Daily Value
Total Fat	65 grams
Saturated Fat	20 grams
Cholesterol	300 mg
Sodium	2,400 mg
Potassium	3,500 mg
Total Carbohydrate	300 grams
Dietary Fiber	25 grams
Protein	50 grams
Vitamin A	5,000 IU
Vitamin C	60 mg
Calcium	1,000 mg

Food Component	Daily Value
Iron	18 mg
Vitamin D	400 IU
Vitamin E	30 IU
Vitamin K	80 mcg
Thiamin	1.5 mg
Riboflavin	1.7 mg
Niacin	20 mg
Vitamin B-6	2.0 mg
Folate	400 mcg
Vitamin B-12	6.0 mcg
Biotin	0.3 mg
Pantothenic Acid	10 mg
Phosphorus	1,000 mg
Iodine	150 mcg
Magnesium	400 mg
Zinc	15 mg
Copper	2.0 mg
Selenium	70 mcg
Manganese	2.0 mg
Chromium	120 mcg
Molybdenum	75 mcg
Chloride	3,400 mg

mg = milligrams
mcg= micrograms
IU= International Units
Source: Title 21 "Code of Federal Regulations" Parts 100-169, April 1, 1995 Section 101.9

Take the Nutrition Label Challenge

Put your know-how to the test and answer the following questions according to the nutrition label on the following page.

Nutrition Facts
Serving Size 2 Tbsp (32g)
Servings Per Container about 16

Amount Per Serving

Calories 190 Calories from Fat 130

% Daily Value*

Total Fat 16g	25%
Saturated Fat 3g	15%
Cholesterol 0mg	0%
Sodium 150mg	6%
Total Carbohydrate 7g	2%
Dietary Fiber 2g	8%
Sugars 3g	
Protein 8g	
Vitamin A 0% •	Vitamin C 0%
Calcium 0% •	Iron 4%

*Percent Daily Values are based on a 2,000 calorie diet

1. How many servings are there in the entire package?

2. How many calories in 2 servings of this food product?

3. How much of your daily percent of iron does one serving of this food provide?

4. By knowing the daily percent of iron in one serving, calculate the amount of iron in milligrams that this product supplies.

5. How much more dietary fiber must you get from other food sources after eating one serving of this food item?

6. How many grams of unsaturated fat are in one serving of this product?

7. Would you consider this food a good source of calcium?

8. Do you think this is an artery clogging food?

9. How many grams of protein are there in one serving?

10. Any idea what this food may be?

Answers to Quiz

1. 16 servings in the entire package.

2. 190×2 servings = 380 calories.

3. 4% Daily Iron.

4. 4% of 18 milligrams = 0.72 milligrams.

5. This product only provides 2 grams of dietary fiber per serving. You'll still need at least 23 more grams from other food sources.

6. Since this product supplies 16 grams of Total Fat, and 3 grams of Saturated Fat per serving, the remaining 13 grams of fat are unsaturated.

7. This product is not a good source of the mineral calcium. At the bottom of the label notice "Calcium 0%." To be considered a "good source" of a nutrient, a food must provide at least 10% of the DV for that nutrient.

8. This food is *not* artery clogging, since it does not contain any cholesterol and the majority of fat is unsaturated.

9. 8 grams of protein in one serving.

10. Did you guess peanut butter?

The Least You Need to Know

➤ The nutrition information provided on prepackaged food labels can enable you to make better informed food choices, and allow you to compare similar food items for the healthier buy.

➤ All of the nutrition information provided is based on one serving size. Check to see how much of a particular food is considered one serving, and if you eat more or less, adjust the nutrition information accordingly.

➤ Try to choose foods that have a big difference between the number of total calories and the number of fat calories. This indicates that a food is not primarily made of fat.

➤ Daily Percent Value refers to how much of a day's recommended amount for certain nutrients are supplied in one serving of a food product. Read carefully and generally stick with foods that have a low daily percentage for fat, cholesterol and sodium, while choosing foods that have a high daily percentage for total carbohydrate, dietary fiber, and all other vitamins and minerals.

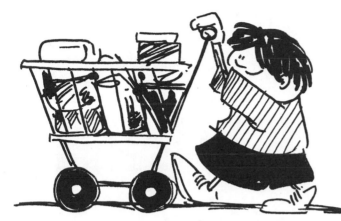

Chapter 10

Stocking Your Kitchen

How many times have you eaten the wrong foods, simply because you didn't have the right foods in your house? Are cookies, cakes, and chips constantly parading on the shelves of your cabinets, or do you furnish the kitchen with fresh fruit and whole-grains? Let's face it, when you are hit with those midday munchies the last thing you feel like doing is driving to a supermarket to buy an apple. More than likely, you're going to grab for whatever is closest to your couch—and who knows what that may be. What about that salad with dinner? No veggies in the house so you'll settle for a prepackaged box of macaroni and cheese. Half the battle to healthy eating is having a variety of nutritious foods on hand, so when the "food-mood" strikes, you're well-equipped to satisfy that growling belly with some savvy food choices.

Take a look in your fridge, pantry, and cabinets to check out what's missing (or shall I say what needs to be removed). Grab a shopping cart and read on, you're about to go grocery shopping!

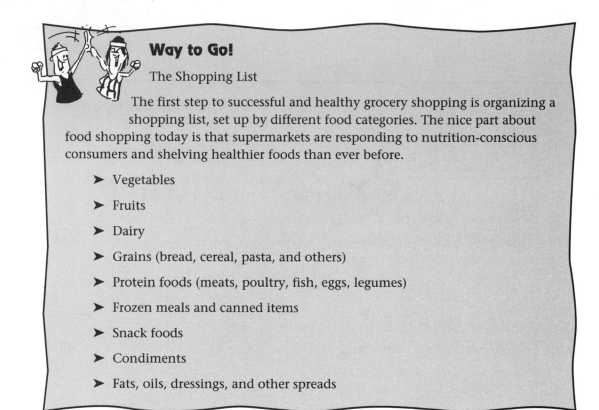

Way to Go!

The Shopping List

The first step to successful and healthy grocery shopping is organizing a shopping list, set up by different food categories. The nice part about food shopping today is that supermarkets are responding to nutrition-conscious consumers and shelving healthier foods than ever before.

➤ Vegetables

➤ Fruits

➤ Dairy

➤ Grains (bread, cereal, pasta, and others)

➤ Protein foods (meats, poultry, fish, eggs, legumes)

➤ Frozen meals and canned items

➤ Snack foods

➤ Condiments

➤ Fats, oils, dressings, and other spreads

Aisle One: Starting with the Produce Section

Talk about a huge bang for your buck! Spend a lot of time walking through this aisle and load up your wagon. Read on to find out why this aisle comes first for nutrition.

Those Voluptuous Veggies

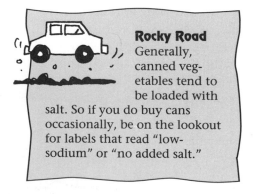

Rocky Road
Generally, canned vegetables tend to be loaded with salt. So if you do buy cans occasionally, be on the lookout for labels that read "low-sodium" or "no added salt."

Vegetables are naturally low in calories and fat, while providing an array of vitamins, minerals, and fiber. Unfortunately, individual bundles of fresh produce do not carry nutrition labels, but you may see posters scattered around the area revealing the beneficial facts on specific items. Rest assured, label or no label, you can never eat too many of these guys!

Most fresh veggies can be judged for freshness and quality by their appearance, so closely examine your produce to avoid any decaying or bruising. Try to be gentle when you lift them up to take a look. (We've all seen those heavy handed shoppers who poke and prod, and usually wind up injuring a perfectly good product.) Another nutrition word of advice is to buy only what you need for the next few days because fresh veggies will go bad if they sit around for an extended period of time.

What if you don't shop so frequently? Or what if you don't have the time to wash and chop your vegetables? Your best bet is to stuff your freezer with the frozen versions. Frozen vegetables come in a variety of combinations (cut, whole, chopped, pureed, along with medley's of premixed veggie concoctions) and all you literally need to do is pop them in a pot to cook. There's no excuse for even the lazy folks! In addition, the freezer keeps the nutrients locked in, so there is no mad rush to eat them before they go bad. What's more, frozen (and canned) vegetables have labels telling all the facts, so take advantage and read.

Way to Go!

"Produce-Smarts"

➤ Buy fresh fruits and vegetables that are in season to keep the prices reasonable.

➤ Examine your fruits and vegetables for freshness before purchasing to avoid bruising and other deformities.

➤ Since fresh produce is perishable, buy only what you need. If you're shopping for an extended period of time, load up on the frozen varieties.

➤ Read the labels on frozen and canned vegetables to make sure there is not a lot of added fat or salt. Read labels on frozen and canned fruits to make sure there is not a lot of added sugar or heavy syrup.

➤ If you're into "super-convenience," buy the prewashed, precut bags of salad, carrots, celery, and anything else offered at your supermarket. Look for premade fruit salads in either the fresh or frozen sections of your grocery store.

➤ Check out the salad bar in your grocery store. This way you can get the exact amount of anything you need, and it's already precut and prewashed for you.

➤ Speak with the person in charge of produce at your local supermarket and ask about unfamiliar fruits and vegetables, then try something new!

Here is a quick rundown on some common vegetables and what to look for when buying fresh selections.

➤ Artichokes provide potassium and folic acid. Look for artichokes that are plump and heavy in relation to size. The many leaf-like parts are called "scales," and should be thick, green, and fresh-looking. Avoid artichokes with any brownish discoloration or moldy growth on the scales.

➤ Asparagus provides vitamins A and C, niacin, folic acid, potassium, and iron. Look for closed, dense tips with smooth, deep green spears. Avoid tips that are spread open or seem to have any mold or decay.

➤ Broccoli provides calcium, potassium, iron, fiber, vitamins A and C, folic acid, and niacin. Look for stalks that are not too tough with compact, firm, bud clusters and that are dark-green or sage-green in color. Avoid bunches of broccoli with a wilted appearance, yellowish-green discoloration, or bud clusters that are spread open. These are all signs of over-maturity.

➤ Brussels sprouts provide vitamins A and C, folic acid, potassium, iron, and fiber. Look for Brussels sprouts with a bright-green color and tight fitting outer leaves. Avoid Brussels sprouts with blemishes or that appear to be wilting.

➤ Cabbage provides vitamin C, potassium, folic acid, and fiber. Whether it's green or red, cabbage can be used in coleslaw, salads, and a variety of cooked dishes. Look for a dense, heavy head of cabbage relative to its size, with outer leaves that display a green or red color (depending on the type). Avoid cabbages with outer leaves that appear wilted or blemished.

➤ Carrots provide vitamin A, potassium, and fiber. Look for smooth, firm, well-formed carrots that have a rich orange color. Avoid roots that are discolored, soft, and flabby.

➤ Cauliflower provides vitamin C, folic acid, potassium, and fiber. Look for compact, firm curds (the edible creamy-white portion), and do not worry about green leaflets that may sometimes be scattered throughout a bunch. Although most grocers sell cauliflower without the outside jacket leaves, in the rare instance that they are left on, a nice green color reveals freshness. Avoid severe discoloration, blemishing, or spreading of the white curd.

➤ Corn provides vitamin A, potassium, and fiber. Although yellow-kernel is the most popular, there are varieties of white-kernel and mixed-kernel corn as well. Look for fresh green husks (the outer covering) and make sure that the silk-ends are free from decay or worm injury. If the corn has already been husked (the outside covering removed) choose ears of corn that are heavily covered with bright yellow, plump kernels. Avoid kernels that appear dried or lacking in color.

➤ Eggplants provide potassium. Look for firm, heavy, dark-purple eggplants (although there are other colored varieties). Avoid any that are shriveled, soft, lacking color, or reveal decay in the form of brownish spots.

➤ Lettuce comes in several varieties: iceberg, butter-head, romaine, and leaf lettuce. It provides vitamin C and folic acid. Look for bright color and crisp leaf texture when buying romaine. For other leafy variations select succulent, tender leaves and avoid any serious discoloration or wilting.

➤ Mushrooms provide potassium, niacin, and riboflavin. Look for closed mushroom caps around the stems, with the underneath gills (rows of paper thin tissue located underneath the caps) colored pink or light-tan. Avoid mushrooms with wide-open caps and dark, discolored gills.

➤ Okra provides vitamin A, potassium, and calcium. Look for bright green, tender pods that are under 4 $\frac{1}{2}$ inches long. Avoid stiff tips (those that resist bending) or pods with a lifeless, pale green color.

➤ Onions are not a significant source of nutrition, but they can certainly enhance the flavor of the foods you eat. With all types (red, white, and yellow) look for hard, dry onions that are free from blemishes. Avoid onions that are wet or mushy.

➤ Peas (green) provide vitamin A, folic acid, potassium, protein, and fiber. Look for a firm, fresh appearance with bright-green colored pods. Avoid flabby, wilted pods, and any sign of decay.

➤ Peppers (sweet) provide vitamins A and C, potassium, and fiber. Although green peppers are the most common, other delicious varieties include yellow, orange, red, purple, and white. Look for firm peppers with deep characteristic color. Avoid very lightweight, flimsy peppers that have punctures or signs of decay on the outside.

➤ Potatoes provide potassium, most B-vitamins, vitamin C, protein, and fiber. Look for reasonably smooth, firm, and blemish-free potatoes. Avoid large bruises, soft spots, and sprouted or shriveled potatoes.

➤ Rhubarb provides vitamin A, calcium, and potassium. Look for firm but tender stems with a decent amount of pink/red color. Avoid rhubarb that appears wilted or flabby.

➤ Spinach provides vitamin A, folic acid, potassium, and fiber. Look for healthy, fresh leaves that have a dark-green color. Avoid spinach leaves that appear wilted or show significant discoloration.

➤ Squash (summer) provides vitamins A and C, potassium, and fiber, and includes several varieties such as yellow Crookneck, large Straightneck, the greenish-white Patty Pan, and the slender green zucchini. Look for firm, well-developed, tender squash. Check for a glossy (not dull) outside, which indicates the squash is tender. Avoid dull, tough, or discolored squash.

➤ Squash (winter) includes Acorn, Butternut, Buttercup, green and blue Hubbarb, Delicious, and Banana, while providing vitamins A and C, potassium, and fiber. Look for squash that is heavy for its size with a tough, hard outside rind. Avoid squash with any signs of decay including sunken spots, bruising, or mold.

➤ Sweet potatoes provide vitamins A and C, folic acid, potassium, and fiber. Look for firm, smooth sweet potatoes with uniformly colored skins. The moist type known as yams should have orange colored flesh, while the dry sweet potatoes have a more pale appearance. Avoid discoloration, worm holes, and any other indication of decay.

➤ Tomatoes provide vitamins A and C and potassium. Look for well-ripened, smooth tomatoes with a rich red color. If you're not planning to eat them within the next few days, choose slightly less ripe, firm tomatoes with a pink/light red color. Only store the ones that are fully ripened in the fridge since the cold temperature might prevent the immature tomatoes from ripening. Avoid tomatoes that are over-ripened and mushy or show any signs of decay.

Those Fabulous Fruits

For a quick nutritious snack, a deliciously healthy dessert, or even part of a creative meal, fruit rules. Similar to its neighbor (vegetables) in the produce section, fruit is naturally low in calories and fat (except for avocado and coconut), while chock-full of nutrients and fiber. Try to get into the habit of regularly replenishing your stash of fresh fruit. Although dried fruit is another tasty option, keep in mind that it is more concentrated in calories since it has less water than its fresh counterparts. Also, beware of canned fruit (and sometimes frozen) with "heavy syrup added"—they are packed with calories and sugar. When buying canned or frozen fruit, read labels and look for key phrases such as "no added sugar," "packed in its own juice," "packed in 100% fruit juice," or "unsweet-ened."

And what about fruit juice? Certainly not a substitute for whole fruit (unless you buy brands with pulp added, it will be lacking in dietary fiber), however, fruit juice does provide nutrients and is clearly a favorable alternative to those sugary drinks people seem to guzzle down WAY TOO OFTEN (colas, sweetened iced-teas, fruit punch). Go ahead and put a couple of juice containers in your shopping cart, but definitely skip the other junk.

Here are some helpful hints when shopping for fresh fruits:

➤ Apples provide potassium and fiber and are available in a bunch of varieties including Red Delicious, McIntosh, Granny Smith, Empire, Washington, and Golden

Delicious. Although each kind differs in seasonal availability, taste, and appearance, some general shopping savvy is to look for crisp, firm apples with a rich color (depending upon the type). Avoid apples with bruising, soft spots, or mealy flesh.

➤ Apricots provide a lot of vitamin A and some potassium and fiber. Look for apricots that have a golden-orange color and appear to be plump and juicy. Avoid apricots that are dull-looking, mushy, overly firm, or have a yellowish-green color.

➤ Avocados provide vitamin A, potassium, folic acid, and fiber. Look for avocados that are slightly tender to the touch if you plan to eat them immediately. Otherwise, buy firm avocados and let them ripen at room temperature for a few days. Avoid any with broken surfaces or dark prominent spots.

➤ Bananas provide lots of potassium and some vitamin A and fiber. Look for firm bananas that are either yellow-green (and will ripen in a few days) or fully yellow and are ready to eat. In general, bananas have their peak quality flavor when the solid yellow color is speckled with some brown. Avoid bananas that are bruised or have a gray appearance.

➤ Blueberries provide vitamin C, potassium, and fiber. Look for plump, firm blueberries that are dark blue in color. Avoid berries that are mushy, moldy, or leaking.

➤ Cantaloupes provide vitamins A and C and potassium. Look for cantaloupes with rough skin that are slightly soft and flexible when you press on the top or bottom, and with a sweet, fresh odor. Avoid extremely hard cantaloupes (unless you want to wait for them to ripen) and any with moldy spots.

➤ Cherries provide vitamin A and potassium. Look for cherries with a dark red color, plump looking surfaces and fresh stems. Avoid cherries that appear dull, shriveled, or dried.

➤ Grapefruits provide vitamins A and C, and potassium. Look for firm, compact grapefruits that are heavy for their size. Do not worry about slight discoloration or skin scars, this usually does not interfere with the quality of taste. Avoid grapefruits that look extremely dull and lack color.

➤ Grapes provide some fiber and come in several color varieties. Look for rich-colored, plump grapes that are tightly attached to the stem. Avoid grapes that are shriveled and soft, or that have brown, brittle stems.

➤ Kiwi fruit provides lots of vitamin C and potassium. Look for plump, slightly yielding to the touch kiwi fruit; this indicates the fruit is ripened. Firm kiwi fruit can be ripened at home by leaving it at room temperature for a few days. Avoid kiwi fruits that are super-soft or shriveled.

➤ Lemons provide vitamin C. Look for firm lemons with a rich, glossy yellow color. Avoid lemons with mold, punctures or a dull, dark yellow coloring.

➤ Mangoes provide vitamins A and C, potassium, and fiber. Look for orange-yellow to red mangoes that are well-developed and barely soft to the touch. Avoid mangoes that are rock-hard or over-ripened and mushy.

➤ Nectarines provide vitamin A and potassium. Look for bright-colored, plump nectarines with orange, yellow, and red color combinations. Nectarines that are hard will ripen in a few days at room temperature. Avoid nectarines that are overly soft, lacking color, or show signs of decay.

➤ Oranges provide lots of vitamin C, potassium, and folic acid. Look for firm, heavy oranges (since this indicates juiciness), with relatively smooth, bright-looking skin. Avoid oranges that are very light (no juice), or have thick, coarse, and/or spongy skins.

➤ Peaches provide vitamin A and potassium. Look for peaches that are firm but slightly soft to the touch. Avoid greenish, hard peaches that are under-ripened and mushy peaches that are over-ripened.

➤ Pears provide potassium and fiber. Look for pears that are firm, but not too hard. The color depends on the variety. Bartletts are pale-yellow to rich-yellow, Anjou or Comice are light-green to yellowish-green, Bosc are greenish-yellow to brownish-yellow, and Winter Nellis are medium to light green. Avoid wilted or wrinkled pears with any distinct spots.

➤ Pineapples provide vitamin C and fiber. Look for pineapples that are plump, firm, heavy for their size, and have a fragrant aroma. Avoid pineapples that appear dull, bruised, dried, or have an unpleasant smell.

➤ Raspberries provide vitamin C, potassium, and fiber. Look for plump, tender berries with a rich, uniform scarlet color. Avoid berries that are mushy or have any mold.

➤ Strawberries provide lots of vitamin C, along with potassium, folic acid, and fiber. Look for firm, red berries that still have the cap stem attached. Avoid berries that have large uncolored or seedy areas. Also avoid strawberries that have a shrunken appearance or any mold.

➤ Tangerines provide vitamins A and C. Look for deep yellow or orange tangerines with a bright luster (indicates freshness and maturity). Avoid tangerines with a pale yellow or greenish color, or punctures in the skin.

➤ Watermelon provides vitamin A and some vitamin C. For uncut watermelons, look for a smooth surface, well-rounded ends and a pale green color. For cut watermelons look for juicy flesh with a rich, red color that is free from white streaks. Avoid melons with lots of white streaks running through pale-colored flesh and light colored seeds.

Aisle Two: Let's Hit the Dairy Section

While I was teaching a fifth grade nutrition class, a young boy raised his hand and asked, "Why don't the supermarkets *only* sell low-fat milk, if the regular stuff is so bad for your body?" I thought, "Wow, wouldn't he make a great president."

In all seriousness, he was absolutely right. Milk products supply you with ample amounts of the mineral calcium (responsible for healthy bones), along with providing protein, several B-vitamins, and vitamins D and A. The problem is that whole milk also contains a lot of saturated fat, which can increase your risk for heart disease, weight gain, and other serious illnesses. What can you do? There is a simple solution—when you are home and have control over the type of dairy that goes into your cereals, recipes, and sandwiches, use the low-fat versions that are available in most supermarkets today. What's more, dairy products carry nutrition labels so you can now utilize your label reading know-how and look for lower-fat milks, yogurts, ice creams, cheeses, sour creams, and so on. Generally, compare two products and see which has a bigger difference between total calories and the calories from fat. This will indicate which brand has less fat relative to the total amount of calories.

Don't throw in the towel if you don't like some of the reduced-fat items—different brands have different tastes. Just try another brand or version the next time you shop. Another thing to keep in mind is that some of the "fat-free" dairy is literally "taste-free" (some brands even resemble plastic). Don't feel you have to suffer with the fat-free if you can't stand the taste, the low-fat dairy is perfectly fine with a mere 3–5 extra grams of fat.

> **Definition**
> **Pasteurized milk:** Milk that has been briefly heated to kill harmful bacteria and then is rapidly chilled.
>
> **Homogenized milk:** Milk that has been processed to reduce the size of milkfat globules so the cream does not separate and the milk stays consistently smooth and uniform.

> **Food for Thought**
> Contrary to its name, *buttermilk* is actually a low-fat dairy product. In fact, buttermilk is simply skim, or low-fat pasteurized milk, with some added lactic acid. The consistency is thicker than regular milk and the sodium is also higher at 257 milligrams per 8 ounces (about double the amount of regular low-fat milk).

Here's your low-fat dairy shopping list. Browse through the section and pick out the items that sound appealing.

- ➤ 1% low-fat milk
- ➤ Skim milk (no fat)
- ➤ Buttermilk

- ➤ Non-fat yogurts (plain and flavored)
- ➤ Low-fat varieties of all cheese
- ➤ Non-fat varieties of all cheese

➤ Non-fat dry milk

➤ Part-skim varieties of all cheese

➤ Evaporated skim milk

➤ Reduced-fat cream cheese

➤ Dry curd cottage cheese

➤ Reduced-fat sour cream

➤ Low-fat cottage cheese

➤ Low-fat/no-fat ice creams

➤ Low-fat yogurts (plain and flavored)

➤ Low-fat/no-fat frozen yogurts

Aisle Three: Getting the Most From Breads, Grains, and Cereals

Here are some shopping tips for buying breads and cereals:

➤ Stick with whole-grain varieties including: whole-wheat, multi-grain, rye, millet, oat-bran, oat, and cracked-wheat (this goes for all types of bread: sliced bread, pita, bagels, English muffins, crackers, etc.).

➤ Although "wheat" bread may sound just as healthy as "whole-wheat" bread, don't be fooled, it's merely a blend of white and whole-wheat flour. For a product to be labeled "whole-wheat" it must be made from 100% whole-wheat flour.

➤ Check the label and choose breads with at least 2 grams of fiber per slice.

➤ If you're looking to save calories, try the whole-wheat, reduced-calorie bread (approximately 40 calories per slice).

➤ Don't forget to check the expiration date on the label!

➤ Take advantage of the fiber that some cereals pack in, and choose varieties that have at least 2 grams of fiber per serving. You can usually (not always) get a sense of whether a cereal has fiber from the name on the box (i.e., Bran Flakes, All-Bran, 100% Bran, Raisin Bran, Fiber-One, Shredded Wheat, and Corn Bran).

➤ Some cereals pack in more sugar and salt than most people realize. Check the *Total Carbohydrates* against the *Sugars* (listed on the nutrition label) to make sure sugar is not a main ingredient. Some cereals contain so much sugar, you may as well be eating jelly beans in milk.

➤ Check the serving size. Some of the denser, heavier cereals only allot a miniscule amount for one serving. Take this into consideration if you plan on eating a normal size bowl. Remember, double the serving size means double the calories.

➤ Don't forget to throw some hot cereal into your cart. Whether you opt for the instant or the kind that requires cooking, stick with "unsweetened" varieties of oatmeal, grits, cream of rice, and cream of wheat. You can sweeten them up with some of the fresh fruit you bought in the produce section!

➤ Most cereals are low in fat with the exception of granola and others that add nuts, seeds, coconut, and oils. Read the label and choose cereals with no more than 2 grams of fat per serving.

➤ Read the list of ingredients on your cereal box and make sure that wheat, rye, corn, or oats are listed first. Items are listed in the order in which they are highest in quantity.

Pasta, Rice, and Other Grains

➤ Pasta is one of those American staple foods that everyone seems to enjoy. What's more, pasta is high in complex carbohydrates, easy to make, and inexpensive. Don't stop at just the box of spaghetti, try the elbow-macaroni, ziti, rigatoni, penne, fusilli, orzo, shells, bow ties, and lasagna noodles. If your supermarket has any whole-grain varieties, throw them in your basket; they're a great source of fiber.

➤ Rice is another excellent source of complex carbohydrates and tends to be a popular standard in many homes. The most nutritious is brown rice, with much more fiber than the white varieties. Next in the nutrition line-up is polished white rice, and last is the instant white rice, with the fewest nutrients of all.

➤ Try some of the not-so-common grains. Pile your cart with couscous, barley, buckwheat, bulgur, kasha, millet, polenta, wheat berries, and cracked wheat. They are all brimming with complex carbohydrates—so jazz up your dinners and impress your family!

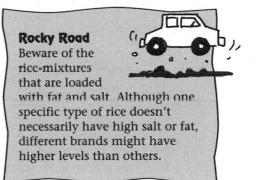

Rocky Road
Beware of the rice-mixtures that are loaded with fat and salt. Although one specific type of rice doesn't necessarily have high salt or fat, different brands might have higher levels than others.

Aisle Four: Best Bets for Protein Foods

When buying beef, pork, lamb, and veal, look for lean, well-trimmed cuts. Meats are graded by the USDA (United States Department of Agriculture) according to their fat content and texture. *Prime* indicates the highest in fat (unfortunately, it's usually the most tender and juicy because of the marbled fat throughout); *Choice* is moderately fatty; and *Select* is the leanest. Lean meats provide lots of high-quality protein, along with iron, B-vitamins, phosphorus, and zinc.

Your leanest beef choices are:

- ➤ lean round
- ➤ lean chuck
- ➤ lean rump
- ➤ lean flank
- ➤ lean sirloin

- ➤ lean tenderloin
- ➤ lean T-bone
- ➤ lean porterhouse
- ➤ lean cubed steak
- ➤ ground beef (extra lean)

Rocky Road
Beware of processed meats that are usually high in fat and salt. If you do buy processed meats occasionally, read labels and compare products. Generally, items that are lower in fat and salt will advertise it somewhere on their cover.

Your leanest lamb and veal choices are:

- ➤ leg of lamb
- ➤ lean lamb chop
- ➤ lean veal chop

- ➤ lamb roast
- ➤ veal roast
- ➤ veal cutlets

Your leanest pork choices are:

- ➤ pork tenderloin
- ➤ loin chops
- ➤ boiled ham

- ➤ pork roast
- ➤ Canadian bacon
- ➤ rib chops

Poultry

Let's not forget about poultry. Poultry can be one of your leanest animal protein sources, but forget about that skin— it's pure fat! You can *buy* poultry with the skin if it's more reasonably priced. You can even *cook* poultry with the skin for some added moistness— just be sure to remove it before eating.

Your leanest poultry choices are:

- ➤ skinless chicken breast
- ➤ turkey breast (white meat, no skin)
- ➤ cornish game hen (no skin)
- ➤ ground chicken or turkey breast (look for no skin added)
- ➤ duck and pheasant (no skin)

Fish and Seafood

When choosing seafood, almost anything goes. Scout the aisle and pick-up anything that looks fresh and appealing. Fresh fish and seafood should have bright skin, bulging eyes (for whole fish), firm flesh, and *no* fishy smell. You may have heard that some fish are fattier than others. It's true, but the amount of fat is so small that all fish and seafood remain great choices nutritionally. In addition, the type of fat found in fish is polyunsaturated (more specifically Omega-3 Fatty Acid), which has been shown to do positive things in the fight against heart disease. What's more, all types of fish supply excellent high-quality protein, along with other vitamins and minerals. So make room in your cart. Let's go fishing!

Your leanest fish choices are:

➤ cod, haddock, flounder, monkfish, sea bass, perch, whiting

➤ tuna, halibut, mullet, red snapper, swordfish, shark

➤ mollusks (abalone, clams, mussels, oysters, scallops, squid)

➤ shellfish (crab, crayfish, lobster, shrimp)

Fattier fish include:

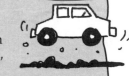

Rocky Road
Try to avoid fish that are smoked, dried, or salted (i.e., smoked salmon or lox). All preparations yield fish that are extremely high in salt!

➤ salmon, albacore tuna, mackerel, bluefish, herring, shad, eel, catfish, pompano

➤ canned fish, like tuna, can also be convenient and healthy. Buy fish packed in water and opt for the lower sodium versions (or wash away some of the salt by rinsing it yourself).

Eggs

Eggs are a good source of high-quality protein, iron, and vitamin A. So what's the problem? I'm sure you've heard it more times than you've wanted: Eggs are too high in cholesterol—about 213 mgs to get technical. Furthermore, there are approximately 5 grams of fat in just one yolk. Not bad if you only eat whole eggs occasionally. Otherwise, start thinking about using only the whites of the eggs, or grab a carton of the egg substitutes (no cholesterol and low in fat) that are generally sold in the frozen section.

Legumes (Dried-Beans, Peas, and Lentils)

Definitely add some legumes to your shopping list. Legumes supply protein, iron, zinc, magnesium, and B-vitamins. Most impressive is that dried-beans, peas, and lentils are the only high-protein foods that provide ample amounts of fiber. Get creative and make a meatless meal a couple of times each week. Look for:

- ➤ baked beans
- ➤ black beans
- ➤ black-eyed peas
- ➤ cannelloni beans
- ➤ garbanzo beans (chickpeas)

- ➤ great northern beans
- ➤ kidney beans
- ➤ lentils
- ➤ lima beans
- ➤ navy beans

- ➤ pinto beans
- ➤ split peas
- ➤ tofu (look for calcium-fortified)
- ➤ vegetarian chilis
- ➤ white beans

Aisle Five: Savvy Suggestions for Frozen Meals, Canned Soups, and Sauces

As mentioned earlier, frozen and canned items can be convenient and tasty. Just remember to read the labels carefully and keep the following tips in mind.

➤ For full frozen meals, always read the label and look for *less* than 400 total calories, 15 grams of fat, and 800 milligrams of sodium.

➤ When choosing soups, avoid the creamy varieties unless you have the option of mixing in your own low-fat milk. Also try to buy soups that say "reduced-sodium," "low-sodium," or "no added salt." Some nutritious selections include: minestrone, garden vegetable, chicken noodle, split pea, tomato-rice, and the lentil-bean combinations.

➤ To cut fat, buy sauces that are tomato or vegetable based. Check the labels and look for brands that have 3 grams (or less) of fat per serving.

Aisle Six: Healthy Snack Cabinet-Stuffers

Most of us love to nibble in between meals. If you plan to stock up your kitchen, do so with these low-fat items.

- ➤ Plain popcorn kernels for air poppers
- ➤ "Lite" or "reduced fat" microwave popcorn
- ➤ Pretzels
- ➤ Baked tortilla, vegetable, or potato chips
- ➤ Raisins
- ➤ Trail mix
- ➤ Flavored rice cakes

- ➤ Fruit and fig bars
- ➤ Low-fat granola bars
- ➤ Lower-fat whole-grain crackers
- ➤ Animal crackers
- ➤ Graham crackers
- ➤ Gingersnaps

Aisle Seven: Condiments to Keep on Hand

The following low-fat condiments can help add pizzaz to your meals. Keep in mind that some of these flavor enhancers are also high in sodium. Salt-sensitive people need to pay close attention to how much of a good thing they are taking in.

➤ ketchup

➤ mustard

➤ jams, fruit preserves, low-sugar spreads

➤ soy sauce, low-sodium

➤ teriyaki sauce, low sodium

➤ balsamic vinegar

➤ cider vinegar

➤ lemon juice

➤ Worcestershire sauce

➤ cocktail sauce

➤ tomato chutney

➤ salsa

Aisle Eight: Smart Buys for Fats, Spreads, and Dressings

When purchasing fats, remember to stick with predominantly unsaturated. Also, opt for the reduced-fat or fat-free versions of the original dressings and spreads. You'll substantially cut down on the fat intake.

Buy 1 or 2 of the following unsaturated oils to have in the house for cooking:

Monounsaturated

➤ olive oil

➤ canola oil

➤ rapeseed oil

➤ peanut oil

Polyunsaturated

➤ safflower oil

➤ sunflower oil

➤ corn oil

➤ soybean oil

➤ Nonstick cooking sprays

➤ Fat-free salad dressings

➤ Low-fat salad dressings (3 grams or less per 2 tablespoons)

➤ Low-fat dips (for all those veggies you bought!)

➤ Soft-tub margarines or spreads

➤ Reduced-fat soft-tub spreads

➤ Butter substitutes (sprays or granules)

➤ Fat-free spreads (go ahead, I dare you)

➤ Reduced-fat mayonnaise

➤ Peanut butter (it may be high in fat, but it also provides a lot of protein. It's a great staple to have in the house)

The Least You Need to Know

➤ The first step to a well-stocked kitchen begins with a comprehensive, healthy shopping list. Make sure to organize your list with individual food categories.

➤ Load up your cart with fresh vegetables and fruit, but only buy what you need since fresh produce is perishable. Frozen and canned fruits and vegetables are good options for people who do not shop frequently—just check to make sure there is not a lot of added fat, sugar, and salt.

➤ Buy low-fat dairy, lean cuts of meat, poultry, and fish, and don't forget about legumes for those meatless meals. Also, look in the freezer section of your market for egg-substitutes; you'll save a lot of fat and cholesterol.

➤ Scout out the grains made with whole-grain flour. When choosing cereals, read the labels and select brands that are low in sugar and provide at least 2 grams of fiber per serving.

➤ Read labels on salad dressings, fats, and other spreads. Opt for products that are "reduced-fat," "low-fat," or "fat-free."

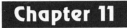

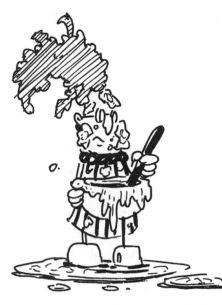

Chapter 11

Getting Down and Dirty with Some Cooking

In This Chapter

➤ Simple cooking modifications

➤ Great recipes for breakfast, lunch, and dinner

➤ Easy-to-make side dishes

➤ Deliciously decadent desserts

Mealtime is the perfect opportunity to bond with your family, converse with friends, relax in private, or impress your date with a knockout dish. So let's go for the gusto, and make this special part of your day even better by preparing a healthy meal. The hardest part is already done, your kitchen is now stocked with the right foods. Now its time to pretend that you're in chemistry lab and experiment with some of these easy-to-make nutritious recipes.

For all you chefs out there, don't be so quick to throw away your not-so-healthy recipes. This chapter offers helpful hints for recipe remodeling; transform your personal favorites into meals that will leave your nutritionist and tastebuds in awe. Go grab some pots and pans and turn on some groovin' music. It's time to get down and dirty with some healthy, imaginative cooking!

The Recipe Make-Over: Remodeling Your Recipes with Simple Substitutions

Skimming the fat in your recipes means more than just using leaner ingredients. It also means using healthful cooking techniques and tools. Here are some quick tips and tricks of the trade:

1. Use low-fat and no-fat cooking methods, like steaming, poaching, stir-frying, broiling, grilling, microwaving, baking, and roasting as alternatives to frying.

2. Get a good quality set of no-stick saucepans, skillets, and baking pans so you can sauté and bake without adding fat.

3. Try no-stick vegetable sprays or 1 to 2 tablespoons of defatted broth, water, juice, or wine to replace cooking oil.

4. Be aware that fat-free or reduced-fat cheeses have slightly different cooking characteristics than their fattier counterparts. For the most part, they don't melt as smoothly. To overcome this, shred these cheeses very finely. When making sauces and soups, toss the cheese with a small amount of flour, cornstarch, or arrowroot.

5. Trim all visible fat from steaks, chops, roasts, and other meat cuts before preparing them.

6. Replace one-quarter to one-half the ground meat or poultry in a casserole or meat sauce with cooked brown rice, bulgar, couscous, or cooked and chopped dried beans to skim the fat and add fiber.

7. Deciding to remove the skin from poultry before or after cooking depends upon your cooking method. Skin helps prevent roasted or baked cuts from drying out, and studies have shown that the fat from the skin doesn't penetrate the meat during cooking. However, if you do leave the skin on, make sure any seasonings you've applied go under the skin or you'll lose the favor when the skin is removed.

8. Skim and discard the fat from hot soups and stews, or chill the soup or stew and skim off the solid fat that forms on top.

9. Use pureed cooked vegetables, like carrots, potatoes, and cauliflower, to thicken soups and sauces instead of cream, egg yolks, or a butter and flour roux. Also, try using soft tofu to thicken sauces.

10. Select "healthier" fats when you need to add fat to a recipe. That means replacing butter, lard, or other highly saturated fats with oils such as canola, olive, safflower, sunflower, corn, and others that are low in saturates. Remember, it takes just a few drops of a very flavorful oil, such as extra-virgin olive oil, dark sesame, walnut, or garlic oil, to really perk up a dish, so go easy.

11. Skim the fat where you won't miss it, but keep the characteristic flavor of fatty ingredients like nuts, coconut, chocolate chips, and bacon by reducing the quantity you use by 50%. For example, if a recipe calls for 1 cup of walnuts, use $^1/_2$ cup instead.

12. Toast nuts and spices to enhance their flavor, then chop them finely so they can be more fully distributed through the food.

13. If sugar is the primary sweetener in a fruit sauce, beverage, or other dish that is not baked, scale the amount down by 25%. Instead of 1 cup of sugar, use $^3/_4$ cup. If you add a pinch of cinnamon, nutmeg, or allspice, you'll increase the perception of sweetness without adding calories.

14. In baked goods, add pureed fruit instead of fat. One of the reasons fat is included in baked products is to make them moist. The high concentration of natural sweetness in pureed fruit will actually help hold on to the moisture during the baking process.

Fat has flavor, but so does fruit. Fat adds liquid volume and moisture to bread or cake batter, but so does fruit. When making this substitution, if the recipe calls for $^1/_2$ cup of fat, simply add $^1/_2$ cup of pureed fruit. Try applesauce in apple bran muffins or cakes. Pureed, crushed pineapple works well in pineapple upside down cake. Here are some other tips:

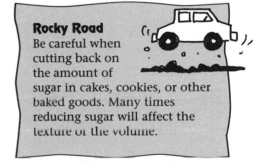

Rocky Road
Be careful when cutting back on the amount of sugar in cakes, cookies, or other baked goods. Many times reducing sugar will affect the texture or the volume.

➤ Dark colored fruits, like blueberries and prunes, are best used in dark-colored batters. Lighter colored fruits, like pears or applesauce, can be added to almost any batter without changing its color. Adding yellow-orange fruits, such as pureed peaches or apricots, can often add an appetizing yellowish crumb.

➤ Pears and apples can be used nearly universally in baking because their taste is very mild and unnoticeable. Apricots, prunes, and pineapple add a much stronger flavor. Bananas and peaches are somewhere in the middle, adding a little flavor, but never overwhelming. And here's a secret: If you don't have a food processor to use to puree your own fruit, try using baby food. It is already pureed, has very mild flavor, and usually is made without sugar.

15. Beat egg whites until soft peaks form before incorporating them into baked goods. This will increase the volume and tenderness.

16. Make a simple fat-free "frosting" for cakes or bar cookies by sprinkling the tops lightly with powdered sugar.

17. Increase the fiber content and nutritional value of dishes by using whole-wheat flour for at least half of the all-purpose white flour. For cakes and other baked products that require a light texture, use whole-wheat pastry flour, available in some well-stocked supermarkets.

18. Vegetables can be fat replacements in other recipes, too. Try:

   ➤ Adding baby carrot puree, roasted red pepper puree, or mashed potatoes to your pasta sauce to replace olive oil.

   ➤ Replacing some of the fat in nut breads or cakes, like carrot cake or zucchini bread, with vegetable purees or juices, like carrot juice or pumpkin puree.

   ➤ Substituting pureed green peas for half the amount of mashed avocado in guacamole or other dips.

   ➤ Replacing fat in soups, sauces, muffins, or cakes with mashed yams or sweet potatoes.

   ➤ Using white potatoes to thicken lower-fat milks in cream soups and bisques.

   ➤ Substituting a layer of vegetables in your favorite lasagna to replace meat or sausage.

   ➤ Topping your pizza with vegetables instead of meat.

   Source: *ADA. "Skim The Fat: A Practical & Up To Date Food Guide,"* 1995.

Top 10 List for Substitutions

1. Use non-fat plain yogurt instead of sour cream.
2. Use 2 egg whites instead of 1 whole egg.
3. Use 1% low-fat milk instead of whole milk.
4. Use ½ the fat that a recipe calls for.
5. Use 3 Tablespoons cocoa powder and 1 Tablespoon oil instead of baking chocolate.
6. Use evaporated skim milk instead of cream.
7. Use fruit purees, fruit juices, or buttermilk to replace fat in a recipe.
8. Use non-fat yogurt or reduced-fat mayonnaise instead of regular mayonnaise.
9. Use diet margarine instead of regular margarine.
10. Use low-fat ricotta cheese or 1% cottage cheese instead of whole-milk cream cheese or ricotta cheese.

Breakfast: Start Your Day with a Bang! Creative Morning Recipes

French Toast a la Mode

Serves three

2 egg whites (or egg substitutes)

$^1/_3$ cup of 1% low-fat milk

$^1/_2$ teaspoon vanilla extract

1 Tablespoon reduced-fat margarine

6 slices of whole-grain bread

1 cup non-fat plain yogurt

1 cup fresh blueberries

Beat the eggs, milk and vanilla in a bowl. Melt the margarine in a skillet over medium heat. Cut the bread into diagonal slices and dip both sides evenly in the batter (made from the eggs, milk and vanilla). Next, brown each side of the bread in the hot skillet by flipping the individual slices. Arrange the finished french toast on a plate (2 full slices or 4 halves per serving)... top with a scoop of yogurt and fresh blueberries.

Nutrient Analysis for One Serving

Calories 231, Total Fat 4 grams

Saturated Fat 0.7 grams, Fiber 7 grams

Protein 13 grams, Sodium 467 mg, Cholesterol 1 mg

*From the kitchen of Carol and Victor Bauer

Egg White-Veggie Omelet

Serves two

8 egg whites

4 Tablespoons low-fat milk

$^1/_2$ cup sliced mushrooms

$^1/_2$ cup sliced onions

$^1/_4$ cup chopped tomato

2 ounces non-fat shredded cheddar cheese

non-stick vegetable spray

pepper to taste

Mix the egg whites together with milk and some pepper, set aside. In a separate dish, place the mushrooms, onions and 2 Tablespoons of water. Cover and microwave the vegetables for approximately 2-3 minutes on high (depending upon how soft you like your veggies). Drain vegetables, and mix in the chopped tomatoes and eggs. Apply non-stick spray to a large skillet, and cook the entire concoction over medium-high heat. When eggs begin to set, sprinkle on the shredded cheese and allow it to melt. When omelet appears cooked but moist, fold over one side and gently lift onto plate. Round-off the meal with some whole-wheat toast and you're set.

continues

continued

Nutrient Analysis for One Serving ($^1/_2$ omelet)

Calories 161, Total Fat 1 grams

Saturated Fat 0.2 grams, Fiber 2 grams

Protein 26 grams, Sodium 445 mg, Cholesterol 1 mg

*From the kitchen of Debra and Steve Beal

Not the Same Old Sandwich Again! "Anything But Hum-Drum" Meals for Lunch

Greek Pasta Salad

Serves four

3 cups uncooked bowtie (or fusilli) pasta

1 cucumber, seed and dice $^1/_4$ inch

3 ripe plum tomatoes, seed and dice $^1/_4$ inch

$^1/_4$ cup chopped red onion

3 Tablespoons black diced olives

2 Tablespoons balsamic vinegar

1 grated lemon zest (the outer peel) and juice

2 Tablespoons fresh chopped mint leaves

olive oil cooking spray

1 small head bibb or butter lettuce

Cook the pasta: Bring 2 quarts of water to a rapid boil over high heat. Add pasta slowly, stirring constantly until all the pasta is in the pot. Bring back to a boil and reduce heat to medium-high. Cook according to package directions or until pasta still has a slightly firm center (about 10-13 minutes). Drain in colander and rinse with cold water.

Make the salad: Combine all vegetables (except the lettuce), vinegar, lemon zest, and lemon juice in a mixing bowl. Toss in pasta and mint leaves and lightly spray with olive oil cooking spray. Toss again. Line 4 plates with lettuce leaves and divide pasta salad among them.

Nutrient Analysis for One Serving

Calories 220, Total Fat 2 grams

Saturated Fat 0 grams, Fiber 2 grams

Protein 10 grams, Sodium 150 mg, Cholesterol 0 mg

Copyright by *Food for Health Newsletter*, 1996. Reprinted with permission.

Open-Faced Tuna Melt

Serves one

1 whole-wheat English muffin, sliced in half

3-ounce can of water packed tuna (low sodium)

2 teaspoons reduced-fat mayonnaise

sliced tomato

2 slices low-fat/low sodium American cheese

Toast both halves of the English muffin and set aside. Drain and mash tuna, then mix with the low-fat mayonnaise. Spread tunafish evenly over both pieces of muffin, leaving the bread open-faced. Place a tomato and one slice of cheese on top of the tuna, on each piece of bread. Put the opened-faced sandwich in the oven until the cheese is fully melted.

Nutrient Analysis for One Serving

Calories 319, Total Fat 7 grams

Saturated Fat 1.5 grams, Fiber 4 grams

Protein 31 grams, Sodium 480 mg, Cholesterol 30 mg

*From the kitchen of Glenn Schloss

Don't Know What to Make for Dinner? Recipes to "Wow" Your Taste Buds

Shrimp and Pineapple Stir-Fry

Serves four

Rice

1 ^{1}/$_2$ cups instant brown rice

1 ^{1}/$_2$ cups water

Stir-fry

canola vegetable oil spray

1 cup assorted sweet peppers (red, green, yellow), dice medium

1 cup sliced mushrooms

^{1}/$_2$ cup snow peas

^{1}/$_2$ cup crushed pineapple, drain and reserve juice

1 cup bean sprouts

continues

continued

$^1/_4$ cup chicken broth

$^1/_2$ Tablespoon cornstarch

1 Tablespoon light soy sauce

$^1/_2$ teaspoon red pepper flakes

12 ounces medium shrimp, peel and devein

Cook instant brown rice in microwave-proof, covered dish for 10 minutes, on medium high power (80%) in your microwave.

Lightly spray a nonstick skillet with canola oil and heat over medium high. Sauté peppers until crisp-tender—about 2 minutes; add mushrooms and snow peas and allow to sauté until crisp-tender—about 2 minutes. Combine chicken broth, cornstarch, light soy sauce and pineapple juice (reserved from drained, crushed pineapple) and add to skillet along with bean sprouts. Bring to a boil, add red pepper flakes and shrimp and cook until shrimp is done—about 1 or 2 minutes. Serve over hot cooked rice.

Nutrient Analysis for One Serving

Calories 290, Total Fat 3 grams

Saturated Fat 0.5 grams, Fiber 4 grams

Protein 23 grams, Sodium 290 mg, Cholesterol 130 mg

Copyright by *Food for Health Newsletter*, 1996. Reprinted with permission.

Swordfish Steaks

Serves three

1 lb swordfish steaks (cut in 3 pieces)

2 teaspoons olive oil

$^1/_2$ bunch fresh parsley

$^1/_2$ bunch fresh cilantro

1 fresh squeezed lemon

fresh, coarsely ground black pepper

Add all ingredients (except the swordfish) into a blender and blend well. Thoroughly coat and marinate the swordfish steaks for 2–12 hours (depending upon how much time you have). Remove steaks from marinade and sprinkle with coarsely ground black pepper to taste. Grill for approximately 4 minutes on each side—grilling time will vary depending upon the thickness of the swordfish and personal preference.

Nutrient Analysis for One Serving

Calories 232, Total Fat 11 grams

Saturated Fat 2 grams, Fiber 0.2 grams

Protein 30 grams, Sodium 142 mg, Cholesterol 59 mg

*From the kitchen of Meg Fein

Jon's Terrific Turkeyloaf with Mashed Potatoes

Serves eight

Turkeyloaf

2 lbs ground lean turkey breast (no skin)

3 slices whole-wheat bread, pulled apart

2 cups whole cranberry sauce

1 whole egg + 2 egg whites

2 carrots, peeled and diced

1 cup onions, diced

1 cup shredded fat-free cheddar cheese

6 crushed cloves of garlic

5 fresh parsley sprigs

Mashed potatoes

5 medium size potatoes, peeled and quartered

2 Tablespoons diet margarine

1 cup 1% lowfat milk

Preheat oven to 350° Mix all turkeyloaf ingredients together in a bowl, then place into a loaf pan. Bake for $^1/_2$ hour...drain off oil.

In a separate pot, boil the 5 peeled, quartered potatoes. When soft (poke with fork), mash them and mix in the margarine and milk.

Now for the finishing touch... spread mashed potatoes across the top of the turkeyloaf and put the combination back in the oven for an additional 30 minutes (at 350°).

Nutrient Analysis for One Serving

Calories 498, Total Fat 4 grams

Saturated Fat 1 gram, Fiber 6 grams

Protein 46 grams, Sodium 325 mg, Cholesterol 122 mg

*From the kitchen of Jon Cohen and Nancy Shapiro

You can find healthy recipes in the following book list:

Cooking Light Cookbook 1996
Oxmore House Publishing
1-800-526-5111

Cook Healthy Cook Quick
Oxmore House Publishing
1-800-526-5111

Low-Fat Cooking for Good Health
by Gloria Rose
Avery Publishing Group
1-800-548-5757

Secrets of Fat-Free Baking
by Sandra Woodruff, R.D.
Avery Publishing Group
1-800-548-5757

Quick and Healthy Recipes and Ideas
by Brenda J. Ponichtera
ScaleDown Publishing
1-541-296-5859

Everyday Cooking with Dr. Dean Ornish
by Dean Ornish, M.D.
Harper Collins Publishers
Available at your local bookstore

Kitchen Fun for Kids
by Michael F. Jacobson and Laura Hill, R.D.
Center for Science in the Public Interest (CSPI)
1-800-237-4874

Quick and Healthy Low-Fat Cooking
edited by Jean Rogers, from the pages of
Prevention Magazine
Rosedale Books
1-800-848-4735

Graham Kerr's Creative Choice Cookbook
by Graham Kerr
Berkley Books Publishing Group
1-800-631-8571

What's For Breakfast—Light & Easy Morning Meals for Busy People
by Donna S. Roy M.S.,R.D. and Kathleen Flores M.S.,R.D.
Appletree Press Inc.
1-800-322-5679

Family Favorites Made Lighter
Better Homes and Gardens
Meredith Books
1-800-678-8091

The American Heart Association Cookbook
Times Books/Random House
1-800-726-0600

Healthy Favorites; From America's Community Cookbooks Prevention Magazine
Rodale Press, Inc.
1-800-848-4735

1,001 Low-Fat Recipes
by Sue Spitler
Surrey Books
1-800-326-4430

Sensational Easy-to-Make Side-Dishes

Sautéed Italian Mushrooms

Serves four

1 10-12 ounce pack of white mushrooms (or 1 lb loose),sliced thickly

2-3 garlic cloves, sliced

chopped parsley

1 teaspoon olive oil

non-stick cooking spray

fresh ground pepper to taste

Spray skillet with nonstick cooking spray and drizzle the olive oil into the pan. Brown garlic cloves over medium-high heat and add sliced mushrooms and chopped parsley. Add plenty of fresh ground pepper (according to your personal taste) and continue to sauté until mushrooms are brown and tender.

Nutrient Analysis for One Serving

Calories 44, Total Fat 2 grams

Saturated Fat 0 grams, Fiber 2 grams

Protein 3 grams, Sodium 5 mg, Cholesterol 0 mg

*From the kitchen of Grace Leder

Cheese-Baked Potatoes

Serves four

2 baking potatoes (about 8 ounces each)	$1/4$ tsp salt
$1/2$ cup low-fat cottage cheese	$1/8$ tsp pepper
$1/4$ cup skim milk	Paprika to taste

Wash potatoes well. Prick skins in several places. Bake at 425° until tender (50 to 60 minutes). Remove from oven; cut in half. Scoop out insides of potatoes, leaving skins intact; save skins. Mash potatoes thoroughly. Add remaining ingredients except paprika, and beat until fluffy. Put mashed potato mixture into potato skins. Sprinkle paprika over the tops. Bake at 425° until heated through and tops are lightly browned (about 10 minutes).

Nutrient Analysis for One Serving ($1/2$ potato)

Calories 140, Total Fat 0.7 grams

Saturated Fat 0.4 grams, Fiber 2.5 grams

Protein 6 grams, Sodium 260 mg, Cholesterol 5mg

©1995, *ADA. *"Skim the Fat: A Practical & Up-To-Date Food Guide."* Used by permission.

Tomato Zucchini Roast

Serves four

3 large, ripe plum tomatoes, dice medium	$1/2$ tsp. Italian spice mix
1 medium zucchini, dice medium	fresh cracked black pepper
1 $1/2$ cups sliced mustard greens	olive oil cooking spray

Preheat oven to 350°. Toss all ingredients together and place into suitable-sized glass or metal baking container. Bake 10-15 minutes uncovered until zucchini is tender. Stir well and serve.

Nutrient Analysis for One Serving

Calories 35, Total Fat 0 grams

Saturated Fat 0 grams, Fiber 2 grams

Protein 2 grams, Sodium 15 mg, Cholesterol 0 mg

Copyright by *Food for Health Newsletter*, 1996. Reprinted with permission.

Decadent Mouth-Watering Desserts

Harvest Apple Cake

Serves twelve

4 cups (1 ¼ pounds) unpeeled, chopped Golden Delicious apples, divided	½ teaspoon salt
	¼ teaspoon each ginger and cloves
1 cup firmly packed brown sugar	¼ cup vegetable oil
¾ cup each all-purpose and whole wheat flour	2 large eggs, lightly beaten
1 teaspoon baking soda	1 teaspoon vanilla extract
1 teaspoon cinnamon	1 Tablespoon confectioners' sugar

Combine 3 cups of the apples and the sugar in a bowl; let stand 45 minutes. Heat oven to 350°. Grease and flour a 6-cup fluted tube pan. Combine dry ingredients in a medium bowl. Combine oil, eggs, and vanilla in a small bowl; stir into the apple-sugar mixture. Stir in dry ingredients and remaining apples until blended. Pour into the prepared pan. Bake 40 to 45 minutes, until a toothpick inserted in the center of cake comes out clean. Cool in the pan on a wire rack 10 minutes; unmold cake and cool completely. Sprinkle with confectioners' sugar.

Nutrient Analysis for One Serving

Calories 213, Total Fat 6 grams

Saturated Fat 1 gram, Fiber 2 grams

Protein 3 grams, Sodium 212 mg, Cholesterol 35 mg

©1995, *ADA. *"Skim the Fat: A Practical & Up-To-Date Food Guide."* Used by permission.

Angel-Devil Smoothie

Serves four

2 cups nonfat plain yogurt

2 cups frozen sliced strawberries

2 chocolate nonfat brownies, broken into small pieces

¼ cup skim milk

Combine all ingredients in blender or food processor. Pulse until all is pureed fine. Serve immediately.

continues

continued

Nutrient Analysis for One Serving

Calories 140, Total Fat 0 grams

Saturated Fat 0 grams, Fiber 2 grams

Protein 8 grams, Sodium 135 mg, Cholesterol 5 mg

Copyright by *Food for Health Newsletter*, 1996. Reprinted with permission.

Banana-Health Split

Serves one

1 Banana, peeled

$1/_2$ cup vanilla fat-free frozen yogurt

2 Tablespoons granola cereal, (low-fat)

Split the banana lengthwise down the middle and line up the two pieces on either side of an ice cream dish. Scoop frozen yogurt in the middle and sprinkle granola on top. You've now got a guilt-free banana split!

Nutrient Analysis for One Serving

Calories 243, Total Fat 1 gram

Saturated Fat 0 grams, Fiber 2 grams

Protein 5 grams, Sodium 65 mg, Cholesterol 0 mg

*From the kitchen of Dan Schloss and Pam Shapiro

The Least You Need to Know

➤ Simple ingredient substitutions can turn your favorite recipes into healthy, low-fat dishes.

➤ Stick with the healthier, lower-fat cooking techniques such as steaming, poaching, stir-frying, broiling, grilling, microwaving, baking, and roasting. Jazz up the flavor with non-caloric spices and seasonings.

➤ Use pureed, cooked veggies instead of cream, butter and egg yolks to thicken soups and sauces. For baked products add pureed fruit instead of butter, lard, and other oils. When a recipe calls for a large amount of sugar, scale it down by 25%.

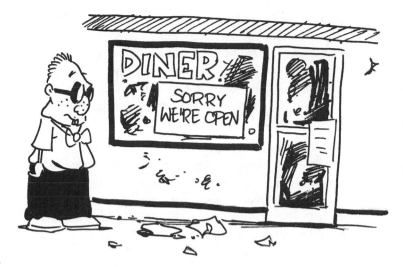

Restaurant Survival Guide

In This Chapter

➤ Dining out healthfully

➤ Becoming a menu detective

➤ Best bets in ethnic cuisine

Don't feel like eating at home? Too tired to cook, or just want to get out and socialize? Join the crowd! According to the National Restaurant Association, Americans spend an average of over $800 million dollars each day on food away from home (that's a lot of moolah). Once considered a luxury for celebrating special occasions, eating out has now become an everyday happening. Whether it be power lunches, the in/out convenience of fast-food, or just plain enjoyment, the food-service industry is growing by leaps and bounds.

Along with convenience and an entertaining environment, restaurants can also provide healthy food. You just need to practice some defensive dining. I admit that sometimes it can be a bit of a challenge, but you certainly do *not* have to throw nutrition out the window just because someone else is preparing the meal.

Common Restaurant Faux Pas

First, the problem of overeating. "Eating out" does not mean "pigging out!" Being in a restaurant doesn't imply you can stuff yourself like a Thanksgiving turkey. (Are you the type who needs to loosen your belt buckle a couple of notches after each course?) I promise it's not the last meal of your life, and there's no need to lick your plate clean even though your stomach is ready to explode. Get rid of that "need to eat my money's worth" mentality and put down the fork when you are comfortably full. And if you can't have extra food staring you in the face, either ask the waiter to take away your plate, or simply pack up the extra food in a doggie bag and enjoy it the following day (not an hour later!).

And what about the actual food choices? What are you supposed to order without wreaking havoc on your waistline and arteries? Making healthy food choices requires a combination of planning, nutrition know-how, and compromise. *Planning* during the day so you can budget your fat and calories. *Nutrition know-how* so you can order the healthier, lower-fat items from your favorite ethnic cuisines. And lastly, the willingness to *compromise* between the foods you should be eating and the not-so-terrific foods you looooove to chow down!

Fortunately, due to the increasing emphasis on health, most places, from fast-food joints to fancy-shmancy establishments, are making an effort to prepare and offer at least a few healthy alternatives. Quite often, you will even notice a *Spa Cuisine* section on the regular menu listing nutrition information underneath the lower-fat entrees. As for the restaurants that do not provide this luxury, don't be shy or embarrassed: Speak up and ask for special requests such as "salad dressing or sauce on the side," "less oil and salt used during food preparation," and "substitute a baked potato or side salad instead of french fries." Remember, good food does not have to wear the price tag of cellulite!

Become a Dining Detective

Go ahead and take on any type of restaurant, I dare you! Transform yourself into the "Colonel Sleuth" of healthy dining and ask yourself (and waiter) the following four key questions before ordering something on the menu.

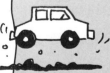

Rocky Road
If you are watching your fat intake, avoid the following high-fat cooking preparations: fried, basted, au gratin, crispy, escalloped, pan-fried, sautéed, marinated (in heavy oil), stewed, or stuffed.

How is the food prepared?

Remember those healthy cooking techniques that were advised for your own personal recipes? The very same methods apply for restaurants. Whether entrees or side dishes, scout out meals that are prepared by grilling, baking, poaching, roasting, boiling, blackening, steaming, broiling, and "lightly" stir-fried. If the menu description does not indicate the cooking technique, ask your waiter/waitress. Don't ever assume that a food is not fried unless it is clearly stated on the menu in black and white.

Are the cuts of meat lean?

Stick with the leaner cuts of meat. For instance, loin, round, flank, shoulder, leg, and extra lean ground beef are the preferred choices when ordering red meat. Chicken and turkey breast are two of the leanest choices to make, and of course, all fish and seafood can be terrific when prepared in a healthful manner. When you do occasionally order steak (notice how I stuck that *occasional* in there), ask if the chef melts butter on top before cooking. Believe it or not, some beef establishments do this to make the meat seem more tender.

What kind of sauces come with your meal?

Ask about the ingredients used for sauces. Generally, avoid hollandaise, butter, cheese, and cream sauces that come slathered over your meal. If you are not sure about something, or it sounds delicious and hard to pass up, get it on the side and enjoy it in smaller amounts.

Food for Thought
Contact your local American Heart Association (or call 1-800-AHA-USA1) for a copy of their pamphlet titled "Savor the Flavors." This informative brochure features tips for choosing healthful meals when dining out.

Are the ingredients loaded with sodium?

If you are on a sodium-restricted diet for medical reasons, it's especially important to avoid entrees and side dishes that are loaded with salt. Stay away from meats and fish that are smoked, cured, pickled, or canned. Sauces, seasonings, and marinades that use soy sauce, teriyaki sauce, dried stock, MSG, or plain old table salt during preparation are off limits! Tell your waiter that for medical reasons you are following a strict low-sodium diet. Can the chef prepare something that will fit into your plan? Most restaurants can be very accommodating when foods are prepared to order.

Q and A

Can you ever just "go whole hog" and order whatever the heck you want without worrying about all the unhealthy ingredients?

Sure you can, but save it for occasional splurges—not everyday habit! In fact, some things are so obscenely scrumptious that if you didn't periodically indulge I'd think you were crazy. So you know that decadent hot fudge, peanut butter, upside-down cheesecake that you constantly dream about in your favorite restaurant... every once in a while—GO FOR IT!

Ethnic Cuisine: "The Good, the Bad, and the Ugly"

Take a quick trip around the world and check out the best bets in French, Italian, Chinese, Japanese, Mexican, Indian, and American cookery. Be adventurous and excite your palate with exotic new flavors. And as they say in the restaurant business, *"BON APPÉTIT."*

Chinese Food

Loaded with vegetables, rice, and noodles, the typical Chinese cuisine offers an assortment of healthy selections. Because most Chinese cooking is done in a wok (stir-frying) there are varying amounts of peanut oil used. The good news is that peanut oil is unsaturated and won't clog up your arteries. The bad news is that excessive amounts of *any* oil can add a lot of fat calories. And as you can imagine, some of the dishes have *startling* amounts.

What can you do if your thighs can't afford those extra fat calories? First, avoid anything fried. If something sounds unclear or suspicious, ask your waiter to explain it. Try one of the steamed versions, or carefully drain off some of the fat in a regular stir-fried entree by removing your portion from the original serving plate drenched in sauce (then transfer it on top of your dish with rice). Another idea, if you are dining with a friend, is to order one dish in sauce, and a second steamed vegetable dish. Mix the two together and you now have $1/2$ the amount of sauce with double the amount of vegetables.

Another problem with Chinese food can be its sodium because a lot of the sauces are high in salt—disaster for salt-sensitive people. Don't be shy, request your food without MSG, and ask if the restaurant offers low-sodium soy sauce for the table. Who knows, maybe the chef will even prepare a special low-salt meal (it can't hurt to ask).

Lower-Fat Foods	Higher-Fat Foods
Hot and sour soup	Egg drop soup
Wonton soup	Egg rolls
Steamed dumplings (vegetable, chicken, and seafood)	Fried dumplings
Stir-fried or steamed chicken and vegetables	Fried wontons
Stir-fried or steamed beef and vegetables	Fried rice
Stir-fried or steamed seafood and vegetables	Egg fu yung
Stir-fried or steamed tofu and vegetables	Cold noodles with sesame sauce
Steamed whole fish	Moo-shu pork
Moo-shu vegetables (with pancake rollups)	Sweet and sour pork
Steamed brown and white rice	Fried chicken and seafood dishes

Lower-Fat Foods	Higher-Fat Foods
Fortune cookies	Seafood with lobster sauce
Lychee nuts	Spare ribs
Orange and pineapple slices	
Low-sodium soy sauce, duck sauce, and plum sauce	

French Food

Many positive changes (nutritionally speaking) have occurred in French food during the twentieth century, from the classic *haute* cuisine that generally uses heavier cream sauces, to the newer *nouvelle* cuisine that uses a lighter and healthier approach to food preparation. Obviously, it's my job to coax you into the latter of the two, but we are human, and classic French cuisine is out of this world! So, during those "occasional" indulgences, ask for sauces on the side, or just tell the chef to go lightly (I guarantee your taste buds will still reach orgasmic heights).

Lower-Fat Foods	Higher-Fat Foods
Steamed mussels	Appetizers with olives, anchovies, or capers
Consommé	Quiche
Endive and watercress salads	French onion soup (with cheese)
Nicoise salads	Cream-based soups
Poached fish	Pate
Steamed fish	Fondue
Lightly sautéed vegetables	Crepes
Bouillabaisse	Brioche
Chicken in wine sauce	Duck or goose with skin
French bread and baguettes	Anything with Béarnaise Sauce
Flambéed cherries	Anything with Hollandaise Sauce
Peaches in wine	Anything with Béchamel Sauce
Fresh and poached fruit	Anything with Mornay Sauce
Fruit sorbet	Anything with the word "cream" or "au gratin"
Wine in moderation	Chocolate mousse
	Creme caramel
	Croissants
	Pastries and eclairs

Indian Food

As with most ethnic cuisines, there are pros and cons to Indian cookery. Beginning with the pros, Indian food emphasizes high carbohydrates such as basmati rice, breads, lentils, chickpeas, and vegetables, all accented with an array of spices. The most common veggies are spinach, cabbage, peas, onions, eggplant, potatoes, tomatoes, and green peppers. The con is that fat can easily find its way into many of the entrees, breads, and vegetable side dishes.

Lower-Fat Foods	Higher-Fat Foods
Tamata salat	Anything made with Ghee (clarified butter)
Mulligatawny soup (lentil, veggies, and spices)	Coconut soups
Chicken or beef tikka	Samosas (fried vegetable turnover)
Tandoori chicken, beef, or fish	Korma (meat with rich yogurt cream sauce)
Chicken, beef, and fish saag (with spinach)	Curries made with coconut milk or cream
Chicken, beef, and fish vandaloo (with potatoes and spices)	Pakora (Fried dough with veggies)
Shish kabob	Saaq paneer (spinach with cream sauce)
Gobhi matar tamatar (cauliflower with peas and tomatoes)	Creamy rice dishes
Matar pulao (rice pilaf with peas)	Fried breads
Steamed rice	Honeyed pastries
Papadum or papad (crispy, thin lentil wafers)	
Coriander, tamarind, and yogurt-based sauces	
Chapati (thin, dry whole-wheat bread)	
Naan (leavened, baked bread topped with poppy seeds)	
Kulcha (leavened baked bread)	
Mango, mint, and onion chutney	

Scrutinize the menu and watch out for the word *Ghee*, which is clarified butter used frequently in Indian cooking. Other oils that are used for sautéing and frying are sesame oil and coconut oil. While sesame oil is unsaturated, it's quite the contrary for coconut oil—arteries beware! If salt is an issue, forego the soups, and ask the waiter to please prepare your meal without any added salt.

Italian Food

Pizza and pasta, could we survive without them? Among my friends and family, Italian seems to be the one type of food that we can always agree upon. (It's amazing how quickly you can get into the mood.) Unfortunately, like every other cuisine, one wrong turn on the menu and you are headed for a nutritional nightmare. For instance, pasta can be a terrific meal if it is ordered with the right kind of sauce; stick with meatless marinara, red and white clam sauce, pomodora, white wine, and a light olive oil. On the other hand, a pasta entree swimming in one of those cream sauces is a big zero (remember, the object is to *walk* out of the restaurant, not *roll* out). Also watch out for super-cheesy entrees such as stuffed shells, manicotti, lasagna, and parmigiana. Hey, don't get depressed, every once in a while we are all entitled to indulge. Just make sure the rest of your day was pretty low-fat and keep these occasional splurges *occasional*—this stuff on a regular basis can be lethal.

Lower-Fat Foods	Higher-Fat Foods
Roasted peppers	Fried calamari
Mussels marinara	Fried mozzarella
Steamed clams	Garlic bread
Lightly marinated mushrooms	Caesar salads
Grilled calamari	Prosciutto
Minestrone soup	Sausage and meatball heros
Pasta with meatless marinara sauce	Calzones
Pasta primavera (not creamy)	Antipasto salad with high-fat meats and cheese
Pasta with red and white clam sauce	Cheese or meat filled ravioli
Pasta with marsala	Meat lasagna
Chicken breast with red sauce	Cheesy vegetarian lasagna
Chicken cacciatore	Cannelloni
Shrimp, chicken, or veal in wine sauce	Baked ziti
	Fettuccine alfredo
Chicken and veal piccatt	Manicotti
Pizza with fresh vegetable toppings	Pizza with pepperoni and sausage
Fresh Italian bread	Shrimp scampi
Fresh strawberries	Chicken or veal scaloppini
Italian ices	Chicken, veal, or eggplant parmigiana
Skim milk cappuccino	Cannoli and other cream pastries
Wine in moderation	Spumoni

Way to Go!

Going Out for Breakfast or Brunch?

Master the following Dos and Don'ts

Do order pancakes and waffles with plenty of fresh fruit and just a touch of syrup. Choose egg-white omelets stuffed with various veggies, Canadian bacon, unsweetened cereals with skim milk, and fresh fruit. Other healthy alternatives: hot oatmeal, cream of wheat and rice (made with low-fat milk), English muffins, bagels, and whole-grain breads with some jam and low-fat yogurt. And to wash it all down, opt for some fresh juice and low-fat milk.

Don't make it a habit to start your day with an unhealthy catastrophe, such as scrambled eggs, bacon, sausage, hashbrowns, cheese omelets, biscuits, croissants, bagels with butter, large cake-like muffins, donuts, pancakes and waffles smothered in butter and syrup, deep-fried french toast, chicken fried steak, or steak and eggs.

Japanese Food

When dining in a Japanese restaurant you really have to go out of your way to eat *unhealthy*. Don't get me wrong, it can be done, but for the most part, the Japanese have really perfected low-fat cooking by utilizing food preparation methods that require little or no oil. Highlighting rice, vegetables, soybean-based foods, and small quantities of fish, chicken, and meat, these meals are artistic, healthy, and most of all, yummy. What's more, once you master the art of using chopsticks, Japanese dining can be a lot of fun. The one drawback with Japanese cuisine is the high-sodium marinades and traditional sauces, which include soy and teriyaki. Ask your waiter if low-sodium soy sauce is available, and to please serve your sauce in a *side* dipping dish.

Lower-Fat Foods	Higher-Fat Foods
Miso soup (soybean-paste soup with tofu and scallions)	Vegetable tempura (battered and fried veggies)
Steamed vegetables	Shrimp tempura
Fish and vegetable sushi	Tonkatsu (breaded pork cutlet)
Sashimi (raw fish served with wasabi and dipping sauce)	Fried dumplings
	Fried bean curd
Hijiki (cooked seaweed)	Oyako domburi (chicken omelet over rice)
Oshitashi (boiled spinach with soy sauce)	

Lower-Fat Foods	Higher-Fat Foods
Yaki-udon	Chawan mush (chicken and shrimp in egg custard)
Yakitori (skewers of chicken)	Yo kan (sweet bean cake)
Su-udon	
Sukiyaki	
Nabemono (a variety of casseroles)	
Yosenabe (seafood and veggies in broth)	
Miso-nabe	
Shabu-Shabu (sliced beef, vegetables, and noodles)	
Sumashi wan (broth with tofu and shrimp)	
Chicken, fish, or beef teriyaki	
Steamed rice	
Fresh fruit	

Mexican Food

If your taste buds cry out for hot and spicy, Mexican food is probably high on your list of favorites. Unfortunately, some of the typical dishes on a Mexican menu can send you straight to nutrition jail! On a positive note, Mexican food does have the potential to be healthy, especially since many dishes are high in complex carbohydrate and fiber—you just need to manage the menu. For example, those fried tortilla chips can be addicting. If you typically gobble down three baskets before your food even arrives they are dangerous! Get them off the table. Stick with cheeseless entrees that include beans, rice, and grilled chicken or fish, and use plenty of salsa in place of high-fat sour cream and guacamole (although guacamole made from avocado is unsaturated, it still has a lot of fat).

Lower-Fat Foods	Higher-Fat Foods
Gazpacho	Tortilla chips
Corn tortillas with salsa	Nachos with cheese
Ceviche (raw fish cooked in lime or lemon juice)	Flour tortillas
Chicken fajitas	Chorizo (sausage)
Enchiladas	Carnitas (fried beef)

continues

continued

Lower-Fat Foods	Higher-Fat Foods
Camarones de hacha (shrimp sautéed in tomato coriander sauce)	Refried beans
Arroz con pollo (chicken breast with rice)	Quesadillas with cheese
Cheeseless burritos	Beef tacos
Grilled fish or chicken breast	Burritos with cheese
Frijoles a la charra	Beef and cheese enchilada
Borracho beans and rice	Chimichangas
Soft chicken taco	Sour cream and guacamole
Chicken tostada	Sopaipillas (fried dough with sugar)
Salsa, pico de gallo, and cilantro	Frozen margaritas and piña coladas
Jalapeno peppers	

American Food

What exactly is American fare? It's not so easy to define these days because most American-style restaurants borrow an assortment of ethnic dishes from around the world. Of course, we *are* responsible for salad bars, steak and potatoes, chicken and ribs, a bunch of sandwiches, and good ole American apple pie, but the typical American menu usually resembles the United Nations.

For example, you can usually expect to find chicken teriyaki from Japan, a stir-fried dish from China, chicken fajitas from Mexico, and a pasta dish from Italy on the spread. The nice part about such a comprehensive menu is that it offers something for everyone (even your finicky kids). Placing heavy emphasis on appetizers, salads, and sandwiches, American food (like other ethnic cookery) can certainly swing both ways. (I'm just talking about healthy versus unhealthy!) When you're in the mood for a sandwich, stick with the unadulterated versions such as turkey, roast beef, and chicken breast. Beware of breads and buns that are pre-buttered before they reach your table (like the buttery grilled cheese sandwich). Ask your waiter to substitute a side salad for those greasy french fries, and stay clear of large salad entrees that pack in more fat than you want to know about (read the descriptions and go easy on bacon, avocado, shredded cheese, olives, and dressings). For standard entrees, look for the usual green flag words (grilled, broiled, and blackened), and check out the desserts listed under thumbs up. You know the routine by now.

Lower-Fat Foods	Higher-Fat Foods
Shrimp/seafood cocktails	Creamy soups
Tossed salads with lite vinaigrette	Caesar salads
Broth and vegetable-based soup	Salads with avocado, bacon, and creamy dressings
Turkey, roastbeef, and grilled chicken sandwiches	Buffalo/chicken wings
Broiled, blackened, or grilled fish, chicken, and lean meats	Fried zucchini and mushrooms
Plain hamburgers, turkey burgers, and veggie burgers	Cheeseburgers
Grilled chicken on top of salad	Grilled cheese sandwiches
Grilled vegetable plates over rice	Philadelphia cheese steaks
Chicken kabobs and rice	Reuben sandwiches
Baked potatoes (with dijon mustard, ketchup, marinara, salsa, or small amounts of butter)	Tuna melts
Pasta with tomato-based sauce	Tuna salad, egg salad, and chicken salad
Steamed or lightly sautéed vegetables	Fried chicken or fish
Frozen yogurt, fruit ice, or sherbet	Hot dogs
Fresh fruit	French fries
Angel food cake	Potato salad
	Fruit pies, cookies, and cakes
	Creamy coffees
	Ice cream sundaes

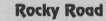

Rocky Road

Don't let the words "Salad Bar" fool you. There are just as many high-fat pickings displayed on the buffet as there are low-fat ones. Survey the situation and load your plate with fresh vegetables, beans, whole-grains, and low-fat dressings. On the flip-side, watch out for the high-fat mayonnaise traps (such as, tuna, egg, seafood, and chicken salads), and take it easy on the creamy dressings, bacon bits, high-fat cheeses, olives, nuts, and seeds.

Fast Food

What has more oil than Saudi Arabia, and is conveniently located on every corner of the world? I'm sure you guessed it, fast-food restaurants.

They may lack ambiance, but fast food is certainly one hopping business! And why not? It's quick, convenient, and cheap. The nice part about fast food today, is that most places offer an assortment of healthy alternatives due to the growing number of nutrition-conscience customers. You just need to learn what to look for. Try your best to keep things simple. Generally, the items with complicated names are laden with high-fat meats and "special sauces." For example, the Bacon Double Cheeseburger Deluxe at Burger King has a whopping 39 grams of fat with 16 grams coming from saturated fat. Be sure to also skip the fried chicken and all sandwiches smothered with cheese...it is not too likely these establishments use low-fat varieties. Also, don't ever assume that fish automatically gets a nutrition gold medal. Did you know that McDonald's Filet-O-Fish (breaded and fried) contains 18 grams of fat, compared to the plain hamburger, which only has nine grams? Carefully scout out what's available before ordering, and stick with the healthier choices below to make the best of your fast-food outings.

Lower-Fat Foods	Higher-Fat Foods
Bagel with jelly	Biscuits and danish
Hot cakes (no butter)	Egg sandwiches
Grilled chicken sandwiches	Sausage and bacon
Plain hamburgers	Cheeseburgers
Turkey burgers	Jumbo burger combinations
Veggie burgers	Fried chicken sandwiches
Vegetable pizza	Fried chicken nuggets
Vegetable salads with lite dressings	Fried fish filets
Chunky chicken salads	Pepperoni or sausage pizza
Turkey sandwiches (no mayo)	Salad bar items with mayonnaise
Lean roast beef sandwiches (no mayo)	French fries
Chicken fajitas	Baked potatoes with lots of butter, sour cream, or cheese toppings
Mashed potatoes	
Baked potatoes with vegetables, salsa, ketchup, or vegetarian chili	Onion rings
	Fried vegetables
Grilled or steamed veggies	Apple pies
Fruit salads and fresh fruit	Milkshakes

Lower-Fat Foods	Higher-Fat Foods
Frozen yogurt cones	Colas
Juice or low-fat milk	Fruit punch
Ketchup, mustard, barbecue, and honey mustard sauce	

Food for Thought

Ellen: Story of a Fast-Food Faux Pas

Ellen, a receptionist for an ad agency, only gets a one hour lunchbreak. Because she doesn't like the brownbag routine (bringing in her own lunch), she quickly runs into one of the three fast-food joints right next to her office: McDonald's, Domino's Pizza, and Wendy's.

At McDonalds she orders a cheeseburger, large fries, and Coke. At Domino's she eats a small pepperoni pizza with extra cheese, washed down with a 7-Up. And at Wendy's she orders a baked potato with broccoli and cheese sauce, with a big, fat Frosty.

Hey Ellen, what's happening? Didn't you read the book? Here are a few lines to help you clean up your act:

➤ At McDonald's, try the McLean Deluxe, side salad with lite vinaigrette, and some orange juice.

➤ At Domino's try a plain pizza with vegetable toppings, a side salad with lite dressing, and a tall glass of water.

➤ At Wendy's try the grilled chicken sandwich on a multi-grain bun, or a baked potato with plain broccoli (or chili), and a salad tossed with lite dressing. Wash it down with some water or juice.

Sky-High Dining

Eating healthy on an airplane can certainly be a challenge. Problem number one, no menu! Sure, they give you a selection of a few things, but everything is already pre-made and there are no substitutions. One option is to call ahead and order one of the "special" meals; Low-calorie, Diabetic, Low-cholesterol, Low-sodium, Vegetarian, Bland, and Kosher (some airlines even provide Hindu, Moslem, and special meals for the kiddies).

If a fruit plate is ever offered (usually with cottage cheese and crackers) grab it (what could they do to fruit?). Unfortunately, the majority of airlines do not provide nutrition information for any of their food, so you're pretty much left in the dark. However, nutrition experts estimate that each meal provides well over 600 calories and is loaded with astronomical amounts of fat (what's worse, they don't even taste good). But I must admit in all fairness that some airlines are putting forth a healthier effort and the inflight meals seem to be getting better. These days you may even be served bagels with low-fat cream cheese, salads with lite dressing packets, rolls with small side tubs of reduced-fat spreads, and pretzels for snacks. Certainly a far cry from Spa Cuisine, but it's a start. Hey, I still say pack your own sandwich, a container of yogurt, and an apple, and watch your neighbor salivate!

Lower-Fat Foods	Higher-Fat Foods
Bagels with jam or low-fat cream cheese	Eggs, bacon, and sausage breakfasts
Cold cereal with low-fat milk and fruit	Fried chicken or fish
Low-fat, low-cholesterol meals	Anything covered in thick sauce
Low-calorie meals	Salty peanuts and chips
Pretzels	Creamy salad dressings
Crackers	Butter packets
Fresh fruit plates	Cakes and cookies
Seltzer and fruit juice	

The Least You Need to Know

➤ Once considered a luxury, dining out has become commonplace for most all Americans today.

➤ Remember that "Eating out" does not mean "pigging out." Don't give yourself the license to overeat just because you are in a restaurant. Eat slowly and selectively, and stop when you are comfortably full.

➤ With the proper planning, nutrition know-how, and willingness to compromise, almost any ethnic restaurant can fit into a healthy low-fat eating plan.

➤ Become a dining detective and examine the menu carefully. Look for lean cuts of meat, poultry, and fish that have been prepared by low-fat cooking methods. Ask your waiter about the type of sauce that accompanies your meal. If salt is an issue, watch out for high sodium marinades.

Part 3
Learning the ABCs of Exercise

Exercise can make you feel more energetic, increase your mental outlook, your balance, your coordination, help to prevent certain diseases, and enable you to look and feel absolutely mahhhrvelous! With all that in mind, this section provides you with the tools and inspiration to get you moving and keep moving. That's right, a crash course on becoming physically fit.

In the following chapters, I'll supply vital information on how to get started on an exercise program that's right for you. You'll hear the lowdown on strengthening your heart and lungs through aerobic exercise, and tips to buff your bodacious bod (try saying that three times fast) through proper weight conditioning techniques. In addition, you'll get the education you need to enter a gym with confidence, and learn how to properly fuel your body—whether for casual exercise or competitive sport.

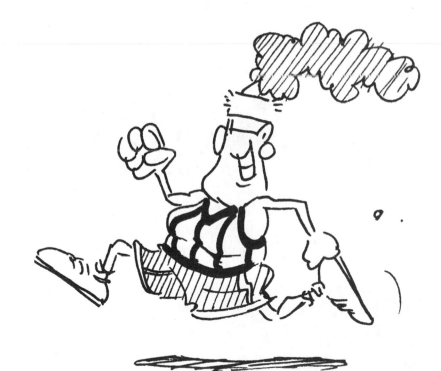

Chapter 13

Let's Get Physical

Throughout history, health professionals (and some hairdressers) have promoted the notion that folks who regularly exercise have better overall health, improved physical functioning, and increased longevity. Even dating back to 400 B.C., the Greek physician Hippocrates (known as the *father of medicine*) addressed exercise in one of his works by writing, "Eating alone will not keep a man well; he must also take exercise." Same thought, different century! So what is exercise anyway? Exercise is formally defined as physical activity that is planned, structured, and repetitive—with the objective of improving or maintaining a level of physical fitness. Simply stated, *exercise whips your body into shape!* So put down the TV clicker, and say "Adios" to the sofa; this chapter is all about *moovin' and groovin'* with exercise.

Prior to plunging your body full-force into an exercise program, take a few minutes to exercise your head. That is, understand the why's, what's, and how's of planned physical activity. *Why* bother exercising? *What* exactly is an appropriate exercise program? And, *how* can you get started? Let's investigate.

Why Bother Exercising?

Simply put, exercise...

➤ Makes you feel better physically.

➤ Improves self-esteem and provides a more positive mental outlook.

➤ Makes you look better and helps to control your weight.

➤ Increases your balance, coordination, and agility.

➤ Helps prevent osteoporosis, cardiovascular disease, and non-insulin dependent diabetes.

➤ Makes you feel invigorated and more energetic.

➤ Strengthens bones and muscle, giving you the functional strength for everyday living.

Before You Begin There Are Some Things to Consider

Hopefully the list above has convinced you that exercising is a big plus. Now let's discuss some strategies that can help you stick with it.

Have realistic expectations. For all you beginners, don't imagine you are going to turn into Arnold Schwarzenegger or Cindy Crawford overnight (unfortunately, this is never going to happen for the majority of us). It's great to have a hero, but understand that people come in all shapes and sizes, and genetics plays a major role in your body make-up and proportion. Rule #1: Exercise is about looking and feeling *your* best—not somebody else's best.

Set reasonable goals for yourself. Plan reachable short-term goals each week that will not leave you overwhelmed, or set you up for failure. An example of a reasonable goal is, "I will work out four days this week, and eliminate all high-fat desserts."

NOT "I will workout two hours every day and lose 10 pounds in two weeks."

Work exercise conveniently into your day. You know the story, unless exercise sessions are planned during realistic time slots, your "work-outs" ain't gonna "work out!" Take into consideration your schedule. Are you a morning person or a night owl? Some people are lucky enough to have leisurely lunchbreaks and can sneak in a quickie during their day (hey, I meant the kind of exercise with your clothes *on*!).

Rise and shine. Studies show that exercisers who workout in the AM, are 50% more likely to stick with it. Sort of like: Get it out of the way before the day wipes you out. What's more, it can also save you an extra shower later on. But, if you have the capacity to endure a grueling day at the office, and then *shake, rattle, and roll* in the gym—more power to you!

Keep it short and sweet. Most people have hectic lifestyles and cannot afford to dedicate hours each day to the gym. And they shouldn't! Each workout should be short and efficient. The *consistency* of regular physical activity is as important as duration and intensity. Without any of these three elements, exercise is simply not effective. Furthermore, people that get carried away usually wind up with injuries or exercise burnout.

What Exactly Is an Appropriate Exercise Program?

An effective exercise program has three main parts: The before, the middle, and the after. The *before* includes a brief warm-up; the *middle*, or bulk of the workout, involves aerobic activity plus weight conditioning; and the *after* consists of a cool down and stretch. Let's take a closer look at each.

Warming Up

A warm-up literally *warms up* the body. By increasing your internal temperature and preparing muscles for the activity ahead, a proper warm-up can help prevent injury to muscles, joints, and connective tissue. What's more, a quick 5–10 minute warm-up will increase the blood flow to the primary muscle groups so that they are ready to rock and roll.

When you think of a warm-up, do you visualize yourself sitting in a straddle position on the floor, moaning loudly while reaching for your left toe (which feels to be somewhere south of the equator)? You're certainly not alone. But let's clear up the facts. Contrary to what most people think, a warm-up does not necessarily involve stretching exercises. Actually, 5–10 minutes of light aerobic activity is an effective warm-up (i.e., biking, rowing, walking, or even marching in place). More specifically, warm up with a lighter version of the exercise you will be engaging in.

For instance, runners can start with a 5–10 minute brisk walk, and swimmers can warm up with a couple of easy, slow paced laps in the pool. Even take a 5–10 minute walk on a treadmill (and include arm circles) before hitting the weight room.

The Cardiovascular Workout: Challenge Your Heart and Lungs

What is aerobics? If you think that aerobics just refers to jumping around to bad disco music, dust off your sneaks—you're way behind the times. The term *aerobic* literally means *with air*. Therefore, the exercises in which your muscles require an increased supply of air (more specifically, the *oxygen* within air) are termed aerobic. Aerobic activity is also known as cardiovascular activity (or cardio) since it most definitely challenges your heart and lungs. Think about this: When you jog, the large muscles of your lower body are continuously working over an extended period of time, and therefore require more than their usual supply of oxygen. Since your heart and lungs are the key players in retrieving and circulating oxygen, it makes sense that they now must go into overdrive to make this increased oxygen delivery. Therefore, in addition to working out the large exterior muscles, aerobic activity also provides one heck of a workout for your heart and lungs.

Normally, aerobic exercise should last for 20–60 minutes, depending upon how much time you have and how fit you are. People who are fit can work longer and harder than those who are not, simply because they can handle the increased demand for oxygen. But for all you beginners, don't let a few discouraging workouts get you down. Doing aerobics is like playing the piano, the more you practice the better you get.

Walking briskly, biking, jogging, stair-climbing, cross country skiing, and yes, aerobic dance are all examples of aerobic activity. Generally speaking, anything involving weights and machines, or a fair amount of standing in place is *not* considered aerobic activity.

What Can Aerobics Do for You?

➤ Burns calories and helps with weight management. (Most people are happy to hear that one.)

➤ Improves the functioning of your heart and lungs, therefore, making you less likely to suffer from serious problems involving these key organs.

➤ Improves your circulation.

➤ Improves your sleep patterns (good news for all you insomniacs).

➤ Improves your state of mind.

➤ Intense aerobic activity can release endorphins, in other words, the "Natural or Runner's High"—*legal in all states, with no nasty side effects the day after!*

How Long, How Much, How Hard?

The following guidelines are set by the American College of Sports Medicine:

➤ *How Long*: 20–60 minutes of aerobic activity per session

➤ *How Much*: 3–5 times per week

➤ *How Hard*: low-to-moderate intensity, or 60–90% of your maximum heart rate (see section below)

Beginners should start with a modest game plan. In fact, beginners need to shoot for 40% of their maximum heart rate and work up from there. As you improve, you can do more activity by going longer, harder, or more frequently. But keep in mind that you should only increase the length, frequency, and intensity one at a time—*not* all three at once. It's the perfect recipe for injuries and exercise burnout.

Are You Working Hard Enough? Let's Check It Out

A couple of easy ways to tell if you are working hard enough during an aerobic workout include taking your heart rate (the number of times your heart beats per minute) and the talk test.

➤ *Testing Your Heart Rate:* Follow this mathematical equation and see if you are working in your training zone (also called target heart rate zone). Generally, your training heart rate falls between 60% and 90% of your *maximum heart rate* (the maximum times your heart can beat in one minute). Although, this formula only provides an estimate, it's a great indication of whether you are working too hard, or not hard enough.

Training Heart Rate Formula: (220–your age) × .60–.90

Let's break it up and take it step by step;

Step 1   Calculate your estimated maximum heart rate (220–your age)

Step 2   Multiply maximum heart rate × .60 for lower range

Step 3   Multiply maximum heart rate ×.90 for upper range

Here's the training zone for a 35-year-old man.

$(220–35) \times .60 = 111$ this is his lower range

$(220–35) \times .90 = 167$ this is his upper range

Therefore, his target zone would range between 111–167 beats per minute. This means if it's lower than 111 he needs to step on the accelerator, and if it's more than 167 he needs to slightly use the brake.

Test Your Heart Rate and Your Math Skills

Now that you know the math, take some time during your workout and give it a whirl. Place two fingers (your pointer and middle finger) on the inside of your wrist (just to the thumb side of the large cords you feel), *or* on your neck (below and off to the side of your chin). Feel for your heart's pulse, and if you can't seem to find it, ask for assistance (don't worry, I promise you are alive!). Once you have located it, use a second hand and count how many beats you feel in a 15 second span, then multiply that number by four. Mission accomplished, that's your working heart rate. Just make sure it falls within the range you have calculated as your training zone (not slower, not faster).

> ➤ *Try the Talk test.* Here's a *much* easier way to tell if you are working at an appropriate level. Can you comfortably carry on a conversation while exercising? If the answer is yes, you are doing just fine. But if you are so out of breath that it's difficult to respond, "Yippee! I'm rich," when someone informs you that you've just won the lottery, you definitely need to slow down. On the other hand, if you can belt out the chorus to "YMCA" by the Village People, you'd better step up the intensity! In the final analysis, you should feel like you are working, but not to the point of a cardiac explosion.

Hit the Weights and "Pump some Iron"

Let's clear something up: Weight training is *not* the same as body building. It does not result in the meat locker-look that many women fear (and incidentally, most men fantasize about). Weight training is about improving muscle strength and muscle tone. For men, who have naturally higher levels of testosterone, it usually does mean an increase in muscle size, *hypertrophy*. On the other hand, women tend to increase the tone without significantly increasing the muscle size. Typically, muscle conditioning utilizes dumbbells and barbells (called free weights), and various types of weight machines (usually referred to by brand names like Cybex and Nautilus).

What Can Weight Training Do for You?

> ➤ Stronger muscles can improve your posture, and help keep your body in balance.

> ➤ Stronger muscles can prevent injuries.

> ➤ Weight training helps to tone, lift, firm, and shape your body.

➤ Stronger muscles can help with your everyday activities such as lugging shopping bags, moving furniture, lifting kids, and so on.

➤ Weight training can help prevent osteoporosis.

➤ Weight training can help to *reshape* problem areas like your sagging arms and your butt. Unfortunately, there is no such animal as "spot reducing," which means zapping off fat from specific body parts. But don't fret, because the combination of eating a low-fat diet and participating in aerobic activity, burns *total fat* from all over your body, and chances are it will eventually come off of your *beastly bulge*.

Your Weekly Weight Training Routine

Your weekly scheduling is just as important as the exercises themselves. It's recommended that you set aside the time for 2–3 muscle conditioning workouts per week, while trying to target all of your major muscle groups (see Chapter 13). A major warning here is *not* working the same muscles on consecutive days. Leave a day of rest in between to allow all those important biological changes to take place. In fact, *resting is just as important as the workout itself.* For instance, if you'd like to work all of your muscle groups on the same day, an effective schedule would be Monday/Thursday/Saturday.

Way to Go!

When training with weights, your first three sets should be 6–15 repetitions, or 70–90% of the maximum weight you can lift.

Another option is doing *split routines*. In this case you can lift more often simply because you split up the muscles being worked over the week. In other words, train your upper body one day and your lower body the next. Or, for those truly gung-ho types, train your chest, triceps, and shoulders on one day, and your legs, back, and biceps on the next. Go ahead and plug in your abdominal exercises whichever day you like. Chest and triceps are involved in pushing-type activities, and your back and biceps are involved in pulling activities; therefore, they should be worked in pairs if you want to split up the upper body workouts. One reason people prefer this type of split routine workout is because they can devote more energy to the select muscles being worked on a particular day.

Q and A

Cardio or Muscle Conditioning: Which comes first?

If you want to do cardio and weights on the same day that's fine. It's also fine to alternate days, whichever you fancy. There is not, as of yet, any definite rule on which you should do first—merely personal preference. Some folks like to be good and sweaty before they hit the weights, while others prefer to get the weight training out of the way and then loosen up with cardio afterwards. The choice is yours.

Cardio and Weight Training: The Perfect Combination

Some people ask which is more important, cardio or weight work? The answer is both. You need the combination of aerobic and weight training for overall fitness. As one of my clients once said, *"Weights make it hard, Cardio gets rid of the lard."*

Cooling Down

The goal of a cool-down is to gradually stop the activity, allowing your heart rate, blood pressure, and body temperature to slowly return to normal. Think about how rapidly your heart is pounding and blood is pumping following an intense bout of exercise—*not* a good time to hit the shower! In fact, stopping an intense workout abruptly is a sure way to get dizzy, and feel terrible after a workout. What's more, cooling down properly can help prevent serious health risks for older or out of shape participants. Take an extra 5–10 minutes and slowly reduce the intensity of the exercise you've been working on. Your body will thank you.

Stretching

Stretching is definitely important for maintaining and increasing flexibility, which in turn makes it easier for you to move around. The best time to stretch is when your body is warm, either after you have done a light aerobic warm-up, *or* more preferably, at the end of your workout following a cool-down period. Proper stretching allows the muscles to relax and lengthen, and it can even help alleviate some built up body tension. What's more, it *may* also aid in the removal of waste products, such as lactic acid. This can prevent injury and improve muscle appearance.

Some general stretching guidelines include:

➤ Always get your blood pumping and body warmed up before you stretch.

➤ Stretch *all* your major muscle groups (not just the one's you think were used).

➤ Hold each stretch for at least 15 seconds—never bounce. You can still feel a good stetch with slightly bent knees.

➤ Only stretch to the point of mild tension, not agonizing pain!

➤ Ask a qualified trainer to show you the correct stretching techniques; there's a lot more to it than touching your toes.

Top Five Exercise Myths

1. *No Pain-No Gain*: What a bogus statement! It is true that both weight training and cardiovascular exercise usually involve *some* type of minor discomfort, such as feelings of slight burning or fatigue, and moderate to heavy breathing. However, pain is an entirely different ballgame. If you feel pain when you work out (particularly joint pain), you are most certainly doing something wrong. (*Houston, we've got a problem!*) Stop exercising immediately and have it checked out with your physician pronto. Pushing through agony can lead to some serious trouble. If it checks out okay, seek the assistance of a qualified trainer; something is probably wrong with your exercise program or technique.

2. *Eating Extra Protein Builds Muscle*: We alreadywent over this one in the protein chapter, but allow me to drive the point home once again. The increase in muscle size, known as hypertrophy, has nothing to do with eating a lot of protein in the diet. Muscles get bigger when you overload them via weight training—*not* Big Macs! The recommended daily amounts for protein has always been, and remains to be 10–15% of total calories, regardless of whether you are Mr. Rogers or Mr. Universe.

3. *Weight Training Will Give Me Bulky Muscles*: After reading about weight training causing muscles to increase in size, it's no wonder most women are running to dump their dumbbells in the garbage. Who wants to get bigger? The majority want to get smaller. Fear not, your lower testosterone levels make you experience increases in strength and tone, without all that increase in size. And incidentally, even men have to have a genetic predisposition to getting bigger. You know how some guys can cut and bulk quickly, while others work their tails off without much result? Stick with a balanced weight training program and I promise you won't wake up looking like Lou Ferrigno with lipstick—a.k.a. "The Hulk."

4. *You Only Burn Fat Working Cardio at a Slower Pace:* This was a myth that got a lot of play back in the 80s with exercise classes actually slowing down the pace to "burn more fat." In terms of weight loss that's just not the case. The crucial factor for losing

weight remains to be *the total amount of calories burned*, and it doesn't necessarily matter whether it comes from carbs, protein, or fat. For instance, a high intensity workout (i.e., jogging) for 30 minutes will burn approximately 350 calories, and a low intensity workout (i.e., walking) for the same 30 minutes will burn approximately 150 calories. So I ask you, which do you think burns more fat? The answer is obviously the higher intensity jogging, because it burns more total calories.

But there is something else to think about. What if you're just starting out and can't sustain a fast pace for more than 5–10 minutes? In that case you're certainly better off doing something at a slower pace for a longer length of time. Again, for the reason that you'll burn more total calories in the end.

5. *Sit-Ups Can Burn Fat Off Your Waist*: Not a chance! Remember, there is no such thing as spot reducing or burning the fat off a particular body part. Fat comes off the body as a whole (through aerobic activity and proper nutrition), and unfortunately, not always in the places you would like it to come from first (such as, "The incredible shrinking bra")! You can buy every tummy-tucker, and blubber-blaster on the market—but the abdominal toning exercises *only* work to strengthen the tissue underneath...they don't zap off that mid-section fat (contrary to what they may say). But look on the bright side, below all the flub you probably have some dynamite looking muscles. Something to look forward to when you lose that outer layer.

How Can You Get Started: Your Personal Plan of Attack

Before embarking on an exercise program, figure out what type of plan will best fit your personality and schedule.

Before diving into any type of exercise program be sure to get the okay from your doctor, especially if you have any type of medical history (such as, high blood pressure, diabetes mellitis, and so on.)

The "What'll Work for Me" Fitness Test

Take a paper and pen and answer the following questions.

1. What type of activities do you enjoy doing?

2. What are your time restraints?

3. Are you a morning person or a night owl?

4. Do you like to work out alone or with people?

5. Do you prefer the indoors or outdoors?

6. What's the weather like in your neck of the woods?

7. Do you want to travel to a facility, or does the privacy of your own home sound more appealing?

8. What is within your budget?

So Many Choices, So Little Time: A Million Things You Can Do to Stay in Shape

Now that you've answered the questions above, you should have a pretty good idea of your personal preferences and limitations. Read through the possible exercise options below and determine which ones are feasible. Be sure to focus on both categories; aerobic (3–5 times per week) and muscle conditioning (2–3 times per week). And remember nothing is set in stone...mix and match often to avoid getting bored or burnt out.

Aerobic Suggestions

Activity	Where you can do it
Walking	outside or treadmill (gym or at home)
Running	outside or treadmill (gym or at home)
Biking	outside or stationary bike (gym or at home)
Swimming	outside or indoor pool at the gym
Skating	outside or indoor rink
Stair climbing	indoor staircase or stair-climbing machine (gym or at home)
Cross-country skiing	outside or machine (home or gym)
Rowing	outside or rowing machine (gym or home)
Aerobic classes:	at the gym or home (using videos)
	low-impact multi-impact step spinning jazz tap funk hip-hop

Muscle Conditioning Suggestions

Body sculpting	classes in the gym or videos at home
Circuit/interval workouts	classes at the gym or videos at home

continues

continued

Activity	Where you can do it
Weight training	gym or home equipment
Weight machines	gym or home equipment
Free weights	gym or home equipment

Food for Thought

Overtraining: Too Much of a Good Thing

Pushing your body more often than the experts recommend (unless you are in an athletic training program), can and usually *does* lead to injuries from over-used muscles, tendons, and joints. What's more, *varying* your exercise intensity and duration is also important to prevent overtraining. For example, some days work hard and long, while other days make it short and sweet. Pay attention to your body's cues (unless of course it's cueing you to sit on the couch and inhale potato chips), and make exercise an enjoyable part of your life.

When Formal Exercise Is Just Not Your Thang!

Not into planned sweat? Only read this far to humor yourself? Well you're not hopeless yet, you can still cash in on some of the benefits. In fact, everyday activities can *also* substantially benefit your health, even if they are done *intermittently* throughout the day. For example, take the stairs instead of the elevator (you say you live on the 25th floor—great!), walk short distances instead of driving the car, join your kids in a game of tag, do some gardening, rake the leaves, shovel the snow, and let's not forget how physical housecleaning can be. Whatever your style, formal exercise *or* increasing plain old daily activity, make your *only* life a healthy and active one.

The Least You Need to Know

➤ Exercise reduces your risk for certain diseases, helps you to control your weight, provides you with strength and vigor for everyday activities, and makes you feel "*grreeeaat*" both mentally and physically.

➤ Three important parts of an exercise program include the warm-up, cool down, and total-body stretch.

➤ Aerobic exercise (also known as *cardio*) is any continuous activity that requires increased oxygen, and therefore, challenges your heart and lungs.

➤ How long, how hard, and how often should you do aerbic activity? The experts recommend 3–5 days each week, for 20–60 minute sessions, at a low–moderate intensity.

➤ Don't forget about your muscles! A proper weight training program 2–3 times per week can increase your strength, reduce the risk of osteoporosis, enhance your posture, and help to reshape your body.

➤ Select activities that complement your personality and time schedule, and vary your routine often so you avoid getting exercise burnout.

Chapter 14

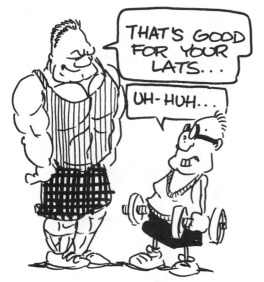

The Gym: Beyond the Locker Room

In This Chapter

➤ Acquainting yourself with the health club scene

➤ Translating gym jargon into English

➤ Popular exercise equipment for cardio and weight training

➤ Your muscles and some exercises to work 'em out

Now that your body is raring to go, you may want to join a local health club. Be sure to prepare yourself for *much* more than a physical experience, because going to the gym can sometimes feel as if you're traveling to a foreign land, or in some instances *outer space*. Between the language barrier, high-tech equipment, scantily-clad thonged women, and members strolling around with biceps bigger than their heads, it's no wonder one may get lost! But don't be intimidated. The gym scene can be terrific. Where else can you have such a tremendous variety of workout choices? What's more, there is always someone available for instruction, encouragement, and motivation. Check out the health clubs in your area, and browse through the basics before hitting the locker room.

Gym Jargon 101

Here's the gym terminology you'll need to hang with the muscle-heads—it's sure to make your conversations with the locals a bit easier.

➤ *"Reps"*: Short for repetitions, meaning the number of times you do an exercise. Usually 6–15 reps are done per set.

➤ *"Sets"*: A group of repetitions. Usually 1–3 sets are done per exercise. (A man working on bicep curls may do three sets of 10 reps. This translates as three full rounds of 10 bicep curls each.)

➤ *"He's/she's ripped"*: A major compliment about a guy or gal's defined physique.

➤ *"You've really got great definition in your...(rhymes with pass)!"*: A tired but effective gym come-on. Sort of gym slang for "WOW" (drool, drool)!

➤ *"Being cut"*: Having well-defined muscles.

➤ *"Being pumped"*: A temporary increase in the size of a muscle due to increased blood flow during exercise.

➤ *"Can I work in?"*: Someone wants to use the weight machine you are using, and they are asking if they can alternate sets with you. Because the gym is usually crowded, it's normal practice to share equipment. For example, you do a set of eight reps and then someone else changes the weight to do a set, then you again, and so on. This only makes sense when you have a bunch more to go. If you only have one more set left, reply, "This is my last set"—gym slang for "Hold your horses big fella, I'm almost done."

➤ *"How many more sets do you have here?"*: Someone is getting antsy to use the weight machine you are on and doesn't particularly want to "work in" with you. This is a polite way of saying, "Are you planning on staying here all day? Perhaps I could order you a cappuccino."

➤ *"Can I get a spot?"*: Basically someone is asking you to help them do an exercise with an amount of weight they are somewhat nervous about using. Politely pass on this one if you don't know how to spot the exercise. Things could get ugly if a bad spot ruins their set (or worse, the weight lands on their head).

➤ *"Juice"*: Slang for steroids. If muscle-heads are said to be "juicing" you can be sure they are not "juicing" with fresh fruits and vegetables.

Resources

Some people decide to hire a personal trainer to help them get into shape. While some exercisers only require a personal trainer for a single "show you the ropes" session, others enjoy continual weekly appointments that help keep them focused and motivated. If you decide to work with a trainer, be very selective with whom you hire because the unfortunate truth is that *anyone* can call themselves a personal trainer. *And, although every former high school football hero fancies themselves a fitness guru, there is plenty about exercise the "has been" athlete does not know.*

Seek out somebody with a BS (better yet, a masters degree) in exercise physiology, physical education, or kinesiology. Or, look for a *"certified"* fitness trainer, which means they have studied for and passed a comprehensive training exam.

Some of the most reputable organizations that provide certifications include:

ACSM (American College of Sports Medicine)

ACE (American Council on Exercise)

NSCA (National Strength and Conditioning Association)

AFAA (Aerobics and Fitness Association of America)

NASM (National Academy of Sports Medicine)

Other comprehensive fitness certifications are offered at various universities.

**Note: Most of these organizations offer a variety of certifications (i.e: aerobic instructor, yoga, and so on). Make sure that your trainer is specifically certified in *personal training* or *fitness instruction*, and that his or her certification is up-to-date.

A Tour of the Equipment

Health clubs are loaded with amazing machinery. With all the high-tech, futuristic equipment that's available, it can almost feel like you are on the set of a *Jetsons* cartoon. *"Hey Jane, how long you been on that stairmaster?"* Take advantage and try them all. Don't get stuck in that "same machine day-in day-out" routine. Swap around from week to week and keep your workouts interesting and fun.

Q and A

Think You May Benefit from Going One-on-One?

Consider hiring a personal trainer if you fall into any of the following categories:

➤ You are completely out of shape and haven't the slightest idea how to begin an exercise program. A trainer can acquaint you with all of the up-to-date exercise techniques and available aerobic and weight machinery.

➤ You are in a *HUGE* exercise rut, and have been doing the same old routine for as long as you can remember. A trainer can show you variations on your day-to-day workout and make exercising a lot more efficient and effective.

➤ You just plain lack the "umph" to exercise on your own. A trainer can help to push, motivate, and whip your butt into shape.

Interview a trainer before you actually set up an appointment to be sure you feel comfortable with his or her workout philosophy, personality, and fee scale. Rates vary tremendously, anywhere from $20–$80 per workout. *They can even run more than $100 if you are looking for that "Trainer to the Stars."*

Get to Know the Aerobic Contraptions

All cardiovascular exercise equipment is designed to get large muscles pumping in a rhythmic fashion—to increase heart rate and blood pressure and burn calories. So what's the best piece of cardio equipment? The answer: Any machine you are really going to use. Pop some jammin' tunes in your Walkman, read the paper, or watch TV (from *Good Morning America* to the *Flintstones*...whatever grabs ya), and you'll be surprised how quickly the time can fly.

Treadmills: Cardiovascular equipment that presents light to moderate impact on your joints depending on whether you are walking or running. Walking on a flat grade is a good starting place for beginning exercisers. As fitness and confidence levels build, you can fool around with increasing the incline and speed.

Stairclimbers: Cardiovascular equipment that provides a very challenging workout with some potential stress to your knees and lower back (listen carefully to your body). This is a more advanced piece of machinery due to the importance of technique, and therefore a base level of stamina and strength is needed to use this machine even on lower levels.

Stationary Bikes: Now they come in two flavors: the upright bike (like a regular outdoors bicycle), and the recumbent bike (legs out in front with high bucket seats lending more support for people with lower back pain). Both types of stationary bikes provide effective aerobic workouts that can give your joints a break because they are non-weight bearing activities. Make sure that the tension is not too high and that the seat is not too low. If you are a beginning biker, ask a trainer to help get you into the proper position for an effective workout. When you are ready to pump up the intensity, play around with increasing your speed before increasing the tension.

Cross Conditioner/Cross-Country Ski Machines: A great aerobic exercise that utilizes the entire body and burns tons of calories without any jarring impact. It's also good for quick warm-ups, because it gets the whole body going. There is, however, one catch: learning the movement can be a bit tricky for some people, and let's just say the term "poetry in motion" takes on a whole new meaning.

Rowing Machines: Another good "total-body" workout (and warm-up machine) without any impact. Be sure to get some pointers on technique; there is an easy way to do it and the *right* way to do it. Obviously the right way requires a lot more energy, concentration, and muscular effort.

Rocky Road

Avoid Exercise Burnout

Do the same thing too much, too hard, or too often, and sooner or later it'll seem staler than a leftover pound cake from 1965. Don't be afraid to vary your activities and change your program. In fact, I encourage it. Try roller blading instead of the treadmill. Try using weight machines instead of free weights. Try an exercise class instead of the Life Cycle. Hey, if you even want to dance around naked, I say go for it (just save it for your house, not the gym).

Become Familiar with the Weight Training Tools

Weight training equipment can be super high-tech (multi-muscle machinery) or super low-tech (a pair of dumbbells and a box). Don't be fooled into thinking that something more complicated means a better workout. That's not the case at all.

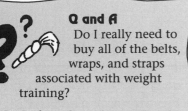

Q and A
Do I really need to buy all of the belts, wraps, and straps associated with weight training?

No. In fact, the only peripheral equipment you may need is a pair of gloves to help protect against calluses

Weight Training Machines: In general, machines are a good starting point for beginners, and those a bit overwhelmed by the gym scene. They can certainly take out a lot of the guess work, simply because you just move from machine to machine. (Adjust your seat, stick in a pin, and you're ready for action!) Several machine variations include weight stacks with pulleys and cords (like Universal and Cybex), metal rod systems (like Cybex and Med-X), cams and chains (like Nautilus), or air pumps (like Kaiser). Just name the nut and bolt and there's a machine out there that has it! Test them all and find the one that you feel most comfortable with.

Free Weights: These, on the other hand, require a fair amount of coordination, strength, and skill since they heavily depend on your balance and body control. Although, weight training with barbells and dumbbells (free weights) may seem significantly harder at first, some people claim free weights yield greater gains than machines. Remember, when embarking on a free weight program, consult at least once with a qualified trainer for tips on proper form and technique. *Bad* habits lead to *bad* injuries.

Resources

Studies report that arthritis sufferers who regularly participate in strength training and stretching programs can greatly improve their balance, speed, and ability to walk, along with reducing joint pain and fatigue. Check it out with your doctor first to be sure there's not too much joint inflammation.

For more information contact the Arthritis Foundation at 1-800-283-7800, and ask about their Aquatics & PACE program (*P*eople with *A*rthritis *C*an *E*xercise).

Learn Your Muscles and "Buff that Bod"

This section provides a quick rundown on the major muscles that conscientious gym folks tend to work out. Of course, your body is action-packed with hundreds more; however, there isn't any reason for you to learn all the others unless you plan to appear on *Jeopardy*. Browse through the list, and become familiar with your muscles *and* the exercises that work them out. Be sure to ask a qualified trainer to personally show you the correct form and technique for each and every exercise.

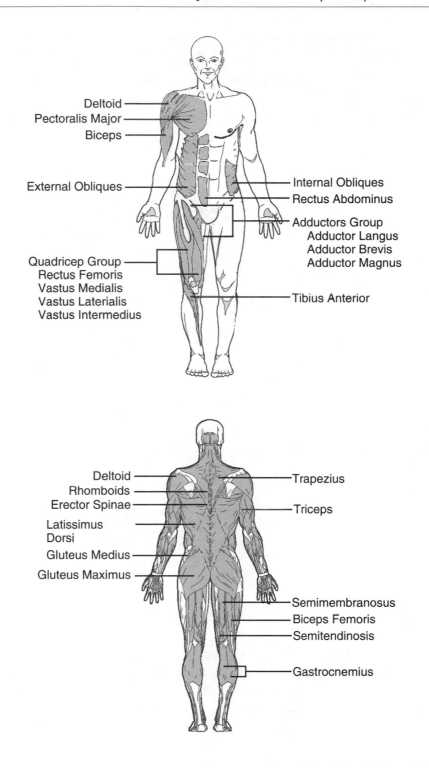

Deltoid
Pectoralis Major
Biceps

External Obliques

Internal Obliques
Rectus Abdominus

Adductors Group
Adductor Langus
Adductor Brevis
Adductor Magnus

Quadricep Group
Rectus Femoris
Vastus Medialis
Vastus Laterialis
Vastus Intermedius

Tibius Anterior

Deltoid
Rhomboids
Erector Spinae

Trapezius

Triceps

Latissimus
Dorsi

Gluteus Medius
Gluteus Maximus

Semimembranosus
Biceps Femoris
Semitendinosis

Gastrocnemius

Gym Slang	Muscle Group	Exercises That Work 'Em
"Traps"	Trapezius	Upper Traps: Shoulder Shrugs Mid Traps: Reverse Flys Seated Rows Lower Traps: Dips
"Delts"	Deltoids	Anterior Delts: Frontal Raises Medial Delts: Lateral Raises Posterior Delts: Reverse Flys
"Midback"	Rhomboids Mid Trapezius	Seated Rows Reverse Flys
"Pecs"	Pectoralis Major	Dumbbell Bench Press Dumbbell Flys Push-ups Dips
"Lats"	Latissimus Dorsi	Lat Pulldowns Seated Row Pulley Rowing
"Lower Back"	Erector Spinae	Lower Back Lifts (on a Mat) Opposite Arm/Leg Lifts on all fours
"Bis"	Biceps	Bicep Curls Supination Curls with Dumbbells
"Tris"	Triceps	Tricep Dips Tricep Pulldowns
"Abs"	Abdominal Group: *internal obliques* *external obliques* *rectus abdominis*	Stomach Crunches Oblique Twist Side crunches
"Butt"	Gluteus Maximus	Leg Press/Squats Hip Extension (with a low pulley cable)
"Outer Hips"	Abductor Group: *gluteus medius* *gluteus minimus*	Abductor Machine Side Leg Lifts (with a low pulley cable)
"Inner Thighs"	Adductor Group: *adductor longus* *adductor brevis* *adductor magnus*	Adductor Machine Inward Leg Lifts (with a low pulley cable)
"Quads"	Quadricep Group: *rectus femoris* *vastus medialis* *vastus lateralis* *vastus intermedius*	Leg Press Leg Extension (also include squats, lunges,and step ups w/dumbbells)

Gym Slang	Muscle Group	Exercises That Work 'Em
"Hams"	Hamstring Group: *biceps femoris* *semitendinosus* *semimembranosus*	Leg Press Leg Curl
"Calves"	Gastronemius Soleus	Heel Raises Straight Leg Toe Presses Straight Leg Heel Raises Bent Leg Toe Presses Bent Leg

The Least You Need to Know

➤ Joining a local gym can certainly be an invaluable tool in your pursuit of that "body beautiful." Take advantage of the tremendous variety of workout choices, and the staffed qualified trainers that can help instruct, motivate, and encourage you.

➤ Some of the terminology used in health clubs can be downright "out of this world." Ask around and learn the lingo so you can converse with the crew.

➤ Some of the popular aerobic equipment commonly found in most gyms includes treadmills, bikes, stairclimbers, rowing machines, and cross-country ski machines. Weight training equipment generally involves either multi-purpose machinery (i.e., Cybex or Nautilus), or free weights (barbells and dumbbells).

➤ Because bad form and technique will most certainly lead to injuries it is strongly recommended that you seek the assistance of a qualified trainer before embarking on any type of program.

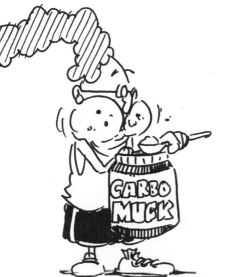

Chapter 15

Sports Nutrition

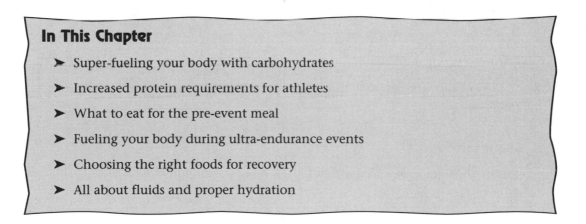

In This Chapter

➤ Super-fueling your body with carbohydrates

➤ Increased protein requirements for athletes

➤ What to eat for the pre-event meal

➤ Fueling your body during ultra-endurance events

➤ Choosing the right foods for recovery

➤ All about fluids and proper hydration

If you've read this far, you know the basics for sports nutrition. Thought you were going to hear about *"potions with power bars,"* or *"instant muscle shake concoctions?"* Sorry to disappoint you, but that's just not going to happen. Contrary to what some people think, there isn't any "magic" ingredient that can help optimize exercise and training. In fact, the very same healthy eating guidelines discussed in previous chapters, *also* apply for competitive sport and casual exercise. You know the story, high on the carbs, low on the fat, and moderate amounts of protein. You may just need to increase your total calories to compensate for the amount continuously burned through activity.

But listen, just because you're familiar with the Egyptian triangle on your cereal box, doesn't mean you should stop reading the chapter now. Believe me, there's a lot more to "sport-specific nutrition" than the basic stuff covers, and this chapter's primed to clue you in. For instance, how does carbohydrate and muscle glycogen work? What's the appropriate amount of protein for athletes in training? How can you properly hydrate before, during, and after an event? What should you eat for the pre-event meal, and what's the deal with ergogenic aids? Stay tuned for a mouthful of information that can help enhance your athletic performance and secure that competitive edge.

Carbohydrates: Fuel of Choice

Carbohydrate is literally the high-octane fuel for exercise, and should provide about 60% of an athlete's total daily calories. To get a bit more technical, you should be consuming 3.2–4.5 grams of carbohydrate per pound of body weight. So where do you fit in? If your sport is pretty low key, and doesn't involve a lot of nonstop running around, you should approximate 3.2 grams. On the other hand, if you participate in a super-endurance sport that involves hours of heavy training each day, you should approximate 4.5 grams.

So what the heck does that mean, anyway?

Math time. Whip out that calculator. Take your weight in pounds and multiply it by 3.2 grams (for low to moderate intensity sports) and 4.5 grams (for strenuous endurance training). Obviously these are two extremes, most exercisers and athletes fall within the middle. In fact, give yourself a range; play around and see where your body feels most vigorous.

For example: Here's the carbo requirement for a 150 pound *elite* runner training several hours each day:

Multiply 150 pounds × 4.5 grams = 675 grams of carbohydrate

Now, let's look at a typical 150 pound health club member, working out at a moderate intensity (approx. 20–60 minutes) 3–5 days a week;

Multiply 150 pounds × 3.2 grams = 480 grams of carbohydrate

As you can see, a more intense endurance exercise program will demand more carbohydrate. But keep in mind, the proportion of carbs, protein, and fat pretty much remain the same as in the previous chapters (55%–60% carbs, 10–15% protein, <30% fat), because in the end, you're taking in more of everything.

Develop Your Own High-Carb Diet

Need to boost your carbs? No problem! Take a look at the wide variety of foods to choose from, and watch how fast you can rack up the grams.

The Starchy Carbs

Generally speaking, breads, grains, and other starchy foods contain approximately 15 grams (give or take a few) of carbohydrate per serving (i.e.; 1 slice bread, or ¹/₂ cup pasta, or 1 serving of cereal). These foods receive top billing for endurance athletes, simply because it's easy to eat multiple servings in one sitting. For instance, a pasta entree can easily total 5 grain servings, and since 1 pasta serving contains about 20 grams of carb, 5 servings supplies a whopping 100 grams of carbohydrate! Clearly this is the reasoning behind marathon runners "packing in the pasta" before the lengthy 26 mile run.

Fruits

Next in the lineup are fruits, also providing about the same 15 grams of carbohydrate per serving (1 medium fresh fruit, 1 cup berries/melon, ¹/₂ cup fruit juice). So why are they second in line? Because athletes looking to load up on the carbs, can more comfortably eat 10+ servings of grain versus 10+ servings of fruit. Remember, fruit has a lot of fiber and tends to fill you up more quickly (you may be "bursting with fruit flavor" in more ways than one). Go ahead and incorporate lots of fresh fruit into your regimen—just don't skimp out on the grains and rely *solely* on fruit—you'll probably get a stomach ache, and more than likely *toot* your way to the finish line.

Milk Products

Milk products contain about 12 grams of carbohydrate per serving (i.e., 1 cup milk, or 1 cup yogurt), and can certainly boost your sum total of carbs together with the starchy foods, fruits, and vegetables. What's more, milk pumps you with calcium, a key ingredient for maintaining those strong, athletic bones.

Vegetables

Veggies provide approximately 5 grams of carbohydrate per serving (i.e, 1 cup raw, or ¹/₂ cup cooked), and are certainly action-packed with vitamins and minerals. Although, veggies alone cannot supply enough concentrated carbohydrate for increased requirements, they can sure jazz up your meals and add tremendous amounts of nutrition to your table.

Common High-Carb Foods	*# of Carbohydrate Grams*
Medium bagel	45 grams
2 slices whole wheat bread	23 grams
1 cup oatmeal	25 grams
1 cup cereal (ready to eat)	16 grams
10 crackers	21 grams
1 cup of pasta (cooked)	40 grams

1 cup rice	35 grams
Granola bar	16 grams
1 ounce pretzels	21 grams
2 fig cookies	23 grams
Power bars	42 grams
Banana	27 grams
Glass of O.J. (8 ounces)	26 grams
Medium baked potato	51 grams
1/2 cup peas	11 grams
1/2 cup corn	17 grams
1 cup low-fat milk	12 grams
1 cup low-fat yogurt (plain)	18 grams
1 cup low-fat yogurt (fruit-flavored)	43 grams
1 cup beans	41 grams

Note that the carbohydrate grams are calculated for serving sizes that are *commonly eaten*, not the standard *single* serving sizes frequently listed throughout the book and on the food guide pyramid.

All About Your Muscle Glycogen Stores

No, the muscle stores are definitely not a chain of shops selling strap-on biceps, but wouldn't that save people a lot of time in the gym. *("I'd like a tricep and 2 huge quadriceps please.")* So what are they, anyway? *Muscle glycogen* is stored carbohydrate in your muscle. To explain further, imagine this: After you eat and digest a meal, the amount of carbohydrate that you immediately need will get used as fuel while the rest (up to a point) will be stored in your muscles for *future* fuel. Athletes who are involved in ultra-endurance sports such as soccer, basketball, hockey, and distance running rely on their high-octane muscle fuel for energy during prolonged bouts of exercise. In fact, between the grueling practice sessions and vigorous competitions, serious endurance athletes are *constantly* depleting and repleting their muscle glycogen stores. That's why athletes participating in high-energy sports require much more carbohydrate-rich foods than athletes involved in

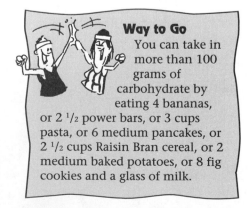

Way to Go
You can take in more than 100 grams of carbohydrate by eating 4 bananas, or 2 1/2 power bars, or 3 cups pasta, or 6 medium pancakes, or 2 1/2 cups Raisin Bran cereal, or 2 medium baked potatoes, or 8 fig cookies and a glass of milk.

less aerobic activity (i.e., golf and archery). But hey, just because you compete in something other than an ultra-endurance sport doesn't mean you can fumble in the carb department. Think about all of the laborious *practice* sessions that wrestlers, divers, or short-distance swimmers put in during the week. Bear in mind, it's not just the actual competition that matters, but the intensity of your training as well.

So what happens if you don't replenish your muscle glycogen stores? Simple: if you run out of glycogen, you run out of energy. You will not be able to sustain high energy activity, simply because the amount of muscle-fuel you have determines how long you will be able to exercise. Just like a car needs a full tank of gas before heading out on a long trip, an endurance athlete requires sufficient "muscle gasoline" to sustain the pace and go the distance. Always tired or rundown? Obviously a vigorous training schedule alone is enough to make you feel that way. You may also want to look into your carbohydrate consumption. Keep a food log and do the math, there could be an easy solution to your problem.

Rocky Road

For all you non-athletes that just decided to browse through the chapter, everyone is *not* a candidate for overdosing on carbs. I know what you're thinking, "Wow! I can constantly pig out on pretzels, pastas, and bagels and it will *only* go into my muscle energy stores." Sure, that's true for incredibly active people who continuously burn buckets of carbohydrate calories (no, casual bowling does not count). However, your muscles can only handle a certain amount of stored carbohydrate, and if you're not utilizing what is already there, you'll likely put on some weight.

What's Carbo-Loading About?

Pasta, Potatoes, and Rice, Oh My! Carbo-loading is just that—loading your body with gargantuan amounts of carbohydrate before an event. Athletes that compete in *extreme* endurance events like marathons and triathlons, can actually manipulate their exercise and eating schedule to help heighten their amount of stored muscle glycogen. You see, during intense, prolonged aerobic activity, your muscle glycogen stores can become severely depleted and cause you to slow down, or worse, drop out. Picture that earlier car running out of gas: putt-putt putt-putt. By super-saturating your muscles with carbohydrate beforehand, an athlete can ensure that their stores are maximally loaded. Here's how it works:

Start this program 6 days before your event

Exercise Schedule		% of Total Daily Food coming from carbs
Day 1	90 minutes	50% carbohydrate
Day 2	40 minutes	50% carbohydrate
Day 3	40 minutes	50% carbohydrate
Day 4	20 minutes	70% carbohydrate
Day 5	20 minutes	70% carbohydrate
Day 6	REST	70% carbohydrate
Day 7	Get out there and kick some butt!	

Personal Protein Requirements

Remember back in the olden days when athletes would eat a huge slab of steak with some scrambled eggs for breakfast, then head off to the field to play some ball? *Protein power, gotta keep up that strength.* Boy, have things changed.

It's true that athletes do, in fact, need more protein than sedentary folks, but being that most people already take in far more protein than the RDA, chances are you're A-OK. Unless you are one of those "carb-o-holics" that live on the "cereal-bagel-pasta" program, you probably get plenty of protein. Perhaps you don't want to waste precious calories on protein? Or, you're trying so hard to carbo-load you forget about the other key ingredients for optimal performance? Whatever your reasoning, *Wake Up, and smell the Gatorade!* Don't you want that competitive edge? Everyone needs protein, especially athletes.

You've already learned the many vital roles of protein in Chapter 5, but let's get sport-specific for a minute. Protein is essential for building and maintaining muscle tissue, along with repairing the muscle damage you endure during hard workouts. Remember, dietary protein does *not* automatically build bigger muscles, *you* build bigger muscles through regular exercise and training. Dietary protein simply allows all your hard work to pay off. Go ahead and take the credit, it had nothing to do with all the extra tuna fish and protein shakes you shoveled in each day.

Below are the recommended daily intakes for protein. Bear in mind that even though athletes have greater protein requirements than couch potatoes, their daily protein proportion still falls within 10–15% of total calories. This holds true because in the end, athletes eat more of everything (especially carbohydrates).

First, find the exercise category you fall into, and then multiply your weight in pounds by the number of grams to the right. After you've done the math and know your personal daily requirements, keep a food log for a week, and tally up your daily protein totals by checking your foods in the chart located in Chapter 4.

Exercise Category	Recommended Daily Protein (grams)
Sedentary folks	.36 grams per pound
Moderate exercisers	.36–.5 grams per pound
Serious adult athletes	.5–.8 grams per pound
Bodybuilders	.5–.8 grams per pound
Growing teenage athletes	.6–.9 grams per pound

Here are some examples;

A 200-pound bodybuilder will need between 100–160 grams of protein daily.

A 150-pound triathlete will need 75–120 grams of protein each day.

A 14-year-old elite gymnast, weighing 92 pounds will need 55–83 grams of protein each day.

A casual 120-pound health club member will need 43–60 grams of protein each day.

Notice that even though the growing gymnast may require more protein per body pound than the bodybuilder, bodybuilders usually (*hopefully*) weigh a lot more, and therefore tend to have greater total protein requirements.

Food Before, During, and After Exercise

Pre-event meals. Let me begin by saying that the most outstanding meal before your sporting event cannot make up for a week's worth of potato chips, french fries, and cookies! With that in mind, study the following guidelines and help make your pre-event meal a "winning beginning."

➤ Make your large meal (approximately 600–800 calories) *at least* 3–4 hours prior to an event. This will provide adequate time for your food to digest. (You certainly don't want to feel weighed down, nauseous, or have indigestion while you're running around on the field.)

➤ Stick with carbohydrate-rich foods and moderate amounts of lean protein. The carbs are both loaded with energy and easy to digest. Avoid eating a lot of high-fat stuff— it takes a much longer time to empty from your stomach and you don't want to have food bouncing along for the ride.

➤ Avoid super high-fiber foods that can cause annoying stomach gurgles, *or* send you running to the bathroom in the midst of a big kickoff.

➤ Also limit the gaseous foods such as beans, brussel sprouts, grapes, broccoli, and anything else you think may give you a gassy stomach.

➤ Liquid meals are also fine, especially if you have the "pre-game jitters" and can't stomach the thought of solid food. Some athletes prefer liquid supplements because they don't leave you feeling as full compared to a large meal of equal calories. In fact, they also leave your stomach quicker than solid food. Personally, I'd rather get my calories from solids, but people are different and the choice is yours.

➤ Also, lay off the salt shaker. As you read in the salt chapter, some people tend to retain lots of fluid, which can lead to puffiness and discomfort.

➤ Never eat something that's completely new before an important competition. *Always* test it during training and see how it settles in your stomach.

➤ Reduce the size of your food intake as you approach the timing of your event. For example: 3–4 hours before you can have a large meal (approx. 600–800 cals), 2–3 hours before you can have a smaller meal (approx. 400–500 cals), and less than 2 hours before you can grab some snacks (bagels, fruit, fig bars, fruit juice, yogurts, and so on).

Ready Made Menu

What time is your sporting event? Which meal will be your pre-event send-off, breakfast, lunch, or dinner? Check out the sample menus and get an idea of the foods you should be choosing. Keep in mind that you should *always* have a well-balanced, carbo-rich meal the night before, especially since on game day you may get fidgety and lose your appetite.

Breakfast: (for a late morning or an early afternoon competition)
Bowl of cereal with low-fat milk
Sliced bananas
Bagel with jam
Glass of orange juice

Lunch: (for a late afternoon or evening competition)
Turkey sandwich on whole-wheat bread
Salad with light dressing
Frozen yogurt with sliced strawberries
Glass of low-fat milk or juice

Dinner: (for an early morning or "anytime the next day" competition)
Grilled chicken
Pasta with marinara sauce
Broccoli and carrots
Fruit salad
2 fig bars
Glass of low-fat milk

Q and A

Is there really such a thing as "winning meals" or "winning foods" that can enhance your performance?

Yes, yes, and yes! You see, if a particular food or meal makes you *mentally* feel at your best, then for you that is a winning meal. Other nutritionists may think I'm crazy but I know firsthand it's true. I grew up as a competitive gymnast. Maybe you've heard of me—I used to go by the name "Nadia Comeniche"—*just kidding.* Every morning before a meet I *had* to have a bowl of oatmeal, 2 slices of toast, and a glass of milk. It was definitely more superstition than anything else, but hey, if it psyched me up, that's all that mattered! So I say if there's a special food or a particular meal that works for you, enjoy!

Fueling Your Body During Prolonged Endurance Activity

Some sports are so lengthy they even require feedings *throughout* the event to help supply your body with glucose when glycogen stores are running low. For example, marathon runners need to take about 40–60 grams of carbohydrate per hour, which translates into a mere (but important) 160–240 calories. Although it's only a minuscule amount, these calories should be spread out over each elapsing hour's time. In fact, your best bet is to nibble on small amounts of fig bars, sports bars, or fruit every 15–30 minutes. Or, make your life simple and just drink one of the popular sports drinks. You can *"hydrate"* and *"carbo-hydrate"* your body at the same time.

Recovery Foods

Now for the last piece of the puzzle. What should you eat for the aftermath nourishment? First, understand that recovery foods are not just for recovering after a competition or game. They're equally strategic following practice workouts as well. In fact, athletes that regularly train long and hard, should focus on replacing emptied glycogen stores, fluids, and potassium lost through sweat on a daily basis. What's more, carbohydrate and fluid repletion should begin ASAP, within 30 minutes after exercise, to help promote a quick recovery time. Sounds unrealistic? Just simply grab for a fruit juice or sports drink while you make the congratulatory "high-five" rounds. Once you are able to focus on a real meal, enjoy whatever you fancy—just make sure to include the following essentials:

➤ Include plenty of fluids such as water, fruit juice, sports drinks, soups, and watery fruits and veggies (i.e., watermelon, grapes, oranges, tomatoes, lettuce, and cucumbers).

➤ Include lots of carbohydrate-rich foods: pasta, potatoes, rice, breads, fruits, yogurts, and so on.

➤ Include moderate amounts of lean protein.

➤ Include potassium-rich foods such as potatoes, bananas, oranges, orange juice, and raisins.

➤ Do *not* attempt to replenish lost sodium by smothering your food in salt, *or* by popping dangerous salt tablets. A typical meal, moderately salted, supplies enough sodium to replace the amount lost through sweat.

Guzzle that Fluid!

Grab that water bottle because you're sure going to need it! In fact, exercise places such great demands on fluid replacement, that proper hydration before, during, and after intense physical activity is critical for top performance. Think about the numerous tasks that depend on fluid: Your *blood* needs fluid to transfer oxygen to working muscles, your *urine* needs fluid to funnel out metabolic waste products, and your *temperature regulating system* needs fluid to dissipate heat through sweat.

You may be thinking, "Okay I understand that blood and urine both require fluid to transport things along, but what the heck does *heat* have to do with fluid?" Here's what happens: When you push your body through exercise, your internal temperature starts to climb. Your body in turn gets rid of this built-up inner heat through the wonderful art of sweating. You may feel wet, gross, and disgusting on the outside, but sweating helps keep your insides within a comfortable working temp so that you may continue on your merry way. If you didn't sweat you'd basically fry up like a scrambled egg.

And now for the fluid connection. In order to sweat you need water—massive amounts of it. In other words, water comes in through your mouth and out through your sweat. It's sort of like fiber, in through your mouth, out through your…(you get the picture). The bottom line is that you need to *continuously* replace the fluid lost through sweat so that you can prevent your body from becoming dehydrated and overheated. What's more, athletes that fail to keep up with their water requirements not only jeopardize performance, but place themselves at risk for serious heat conditions (i.e, heat cramps, heat exhaustion, and heat stroke).

Guidelines for Proper Hydration

Unfortunately for athletes, the thirst mechanism is an unreliable indicator. By the time you feel thirsty, you could already be on your way to dehydration; *plus* the amount of fluid that quenches your thirst may not be enough to quench your body. To ensure adequate hydration, you need to follow a drinking time schedule. Here's what's recommended:

➤ 16 ounces (or 2 cups) 2 hours prior to exercise

➤ 8–16 ounces (or 1–2 cups) 15–30 minutes *before* exercise

➤ 4–8 ounces (or ¹/₂–1 cup) every 15 minutes *during* exercise

➤ 16 ounces (or 2 cups) for every pound lost *after* exercise

How to Check Your Hydration Status

The Pre/Post Scale Test

Hop on the scale and weigh yourself before and after you exercise. For each pound of fluid lost (it's just fluid, *not* fat) drink 2 cups of water (or other fluid) to properly *rehydrate* your body. You don't necessarily have to gulp it all down at once, just make sure that you're fully hydrated by the next day. For example, a soccer player weighs 165 pounds before the game and 162 pounds after the game. Therefore he must drink 6 cups of water to replace the 3 pounds of lost fluid.

Check your urine

The color of your urine is also a good indicator of hydration status. If your urine is voluminous, and clear to pale yellow, you're doing just fine. On the other hand, if your urine is dark and concentrated, keep chugging that fluid, you've got a ways to go!

Rocky Road
Alcohol, coffee, and tea act as *diuretics*, substances that cause you to urinate and therefore lose water. Remember the object is to replace water losses *not* add insult to injury by drinking something that would make you lose it.

Sports Drinks versus Water

Plain old H₂0 is cheap, effective, and just fine for most athletes, but there are some instances that you'll benefit from the added carbohydrate in a sports drink (i.e., Gatorade, PowerAde, All Sport, and so on.). So when should you spring for the loaded stuff? When continuous exercise lasts longer than 60 minutes, *or* when you're exercising in extremely hot weather. You see, where the water can provide straight hydration, the sports drinks can also provide some electrolytes and carbohydrate—just enough to keep you moving and grooving during those exceptionally long *or* hot workouts.

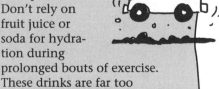

Rocky Road
Don't rely on fruit juice or soda for hydration during prolonged bouts of exercise. These drinks are far too concentrated with calories, and therefore take a long time to empty from your stomach. Sports drinks on the other hand, are special dilute formulas that leave your stomach as rapidly as plain water.

What's the Story on Ergogenic Aids?

Depending upon the positioning of the moon and the pull of the tides (and the color of your father's tie), people make outrageous claims regarding substances that can help enhance performance. The word *ergogenic* literally means "work producing" and, unfortunately, there are constantly cockamamie advertisements claiming to sell nutritional pills and potions that can beef up performance. Let's set the record straight: There are only a few scientifically sound nutritional ergogenic aids, including a proper carbohydrate diet, carbo-loading, and sports drinks. The key to a competitive edge is a well-trained body, a determined soul, and the right equipment. Remember, if it sounds too good to be true, it probably is.

Food for Thought

The Food Obsessed Athlete

It's both sad and ironic to think that the very same people we consider health heroes may be fighting life threatening battles with food. In fact, some athletes can get so caught up in achieving that "perfect body," that they jeopardize both athletic performance, and in some instances, their lives.

I frequently see clients who are competitive gymnasts, ballet dancers, marathon runners, divers, figure skaters, and wrestlers. Notice the connection? All are involved in sports that emphasize low body weights. For more information see Chapter 24.

The Least You Need to Know

➤ Athletes need to primarily focus on eating carbohydrate-rich foods such as grains, pasta, rice, fruits, and veggies. Carbohydrates supply energy for both grueling practice sessions and competitions.

➤ Athletes have greater daily protein requirements than sedentary folks. They require .5–.8 grams protein per pound of body weight.

➤ Proper hydration is essential for maintaining prolonged activity *and* for optimal performance. Water is the perfect fluid replacement for exercise lasting under 60 minutes. However, the ultra endurance athletes, and athletes exercising in extremely hot weather, will benefit from the added carbohydrate and electrolyte content in the popular sports drinks.

➤ Don't be misled by ads claiming to sell enhancers in the shape of a pill. The way to optimize performance is by eating smart and training hard!

Part 4
Nutrition Sidelines

Some people choose not to eat certain foods, while others must avoid specific foods due to medical conditions.

This section provides a complete guide on vegetarianism for that ever-growing "meat-less crowd," along with discussing the foods that may ail you, food allergies, food intolerances, and other food-related hypersensitivities. So whether you purely feast on plants, or bolt for the bathroom after ingesting cheese, stayed tuned.

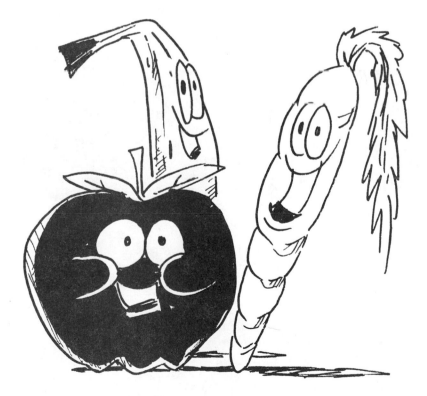

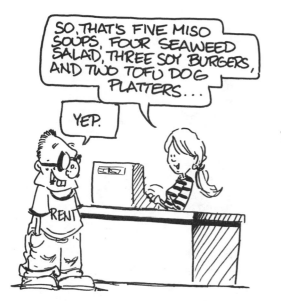

Chapter 16

"Vegging Out"

In This Chapter

➤ Reasons to go vegetarian

➤ What are vegans, lacto-vegetarians, and ovolacto-vegetarians?

➤ Keeping up with your calcium, B-12, and zinc requirements

➤ Great vegetarian protein and iron sources

➤ What's soy protein all about?

➤ Meatless recipes to tantalize your taste buds

Vegetarian diets are becoming increasingly popular with more and more Americans jumping on the "tofu bandwagon." Like every other prudent diet, people following vegetarian food plans must eat well-balanced, varied meals and include fruits, vegetables, nuts, seeds, low-fat dairy (depending upon your vegetarian restrictions), legumes, and plenty of whole grain products. Although typically a vegetarian eating plan tends to be super low in saturated fat and cholesterol, it's not automatically low in *total* fat and sugar. Therefore, *veg-heads* like *meat-heads*, also need to limit their intake of fatty foods, oils, spreads, and sweets.

Food for Thought

A vegetarian diet, when properly followed, can be one of the healthiest diets out there. Benefits of the vegetarian diet include:

➤ Decreased obesity. Vegans are rarely obese and on the average, ovolacto-vegetarians are leaner than those who eat meat. However, being vegetarian doesn't guarantee a slim figure. If you eat foods that are high in fat you can consume as many or more calories than meat eaters.

➤ Less risk of CHD. Vegetarians tend to have lower blood cholesterol levels and diets with lower overall saturated fat content.

➤ Lower rates of hypertension. The reason for this is still unknown, but researchers think that it may be related to increased potassium, magnesium, polyunsaturated fat, and increased fiber intake. All the same, more research is still needed to determine if the diet itself has anything to do with the lower levels.

The Vegetarian Food Guide Pyramid

Similar to the Food Guide Pyramid used as the mainstream standard, the vegetarian version provides recommended guidelines for the "meatless" population.

Refer back to Chapter 1 to find out what a serving size equals for the grain group, vegetable group, fruit group, and dairy group. As for the special vegetarian protein category titled "Legume, Nut, Seed, and Meat Alternative Group," here's the deal on portion sizes;

1 serving equals = $^1/_2$ cup cooked beans or peas, or

$^1/_2$ cup tofu, or

$^1/_4$ cup seeds, or

$^1/_4$ cup (1 ounce) nuts, or

2 Tablespoons nut butter, or

$^1/_4$ cup meat alternative, or

2 eggs (preferably whites)

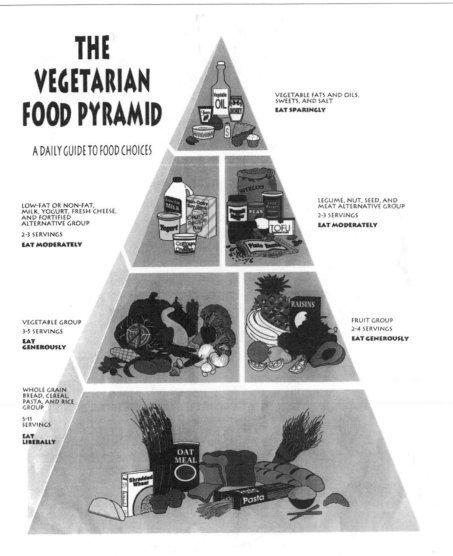

THE VEGETARIAN FOOD PYRAMID

A DAILY GUIDE TO FOOD CHOICES

VEGETABLE FATS AND OILS, SWEETS, AND SALT
EAT SPARINGLY

LOW-FAT OR NON-FAT, MILK, YOGURT, FRESH CHEESE, AND FORTIFIED ALTERNATIVE GROUP
2-3 SERVINGS
EAT MODERATELY

LEGUME, NUT, SEED, AND MEAT ALTERNATIVE GROUP
2-3 SERVINGS
EAT MODERATELY

VEGETABLE GROUP
3-5 SERVINGS
EAT GENEROUSLY

FRUIT GROUP
2-4 SERVINGS
EAT GENEROUSLY

WHOLE GRAIN BREAD, CEREAL, PASTA, AND RICE GROUP
5-11 SERVINGS
EAT LIBERALLY

Source: from The Health Connection©, 1-800-548-8700. To order poster or handouts, please call the toll free number above or (301)790-9735.

The Various Types of Vegetarians

Vegetarian eating covers broad territory and can run the gamut from people who avoid *all* animal products to people who simply refrain from eating a few select animal foods. Here's a look at the assortment of vegetarian-style eaters.

Vegans   This is the strictest type of vegetarian (sort of the Pope of all vegetarians). Vegans abstain from eating or using *all* animal products, from eating meat, dairy, and eggs, to wearing wool, silk, or leather. If you're a vegan you'll need to be extra responsible about getting adequate protein, iron, calcium, vitamin D, vitamin B-12, and zinc.

Lacto-vegetarians   This group eliminates meat and eggs but includes all dairy products.

Ovolacto-vegetarians   This group eliminates all meat (red meat, poultry, fish, and seafood), however, they do include dairy products and eggs.

Semi-vegetarians   This group does not eat red meat, but eats most chicken, turkey, and fish, along with all dairy and eggs.

"Psuedo"-vegetarians   This group will not eat meat on the days they decide they're vegetarian, but will, however, inhale hamburgers and steak sandwiches when they get a craving.

Food for Thought

Tips for the Dining Out Vegetarian

➤ Whenever possible, try to choose a restaurant with a vegetarian cuisine. Scout out your neighborhood and discover what's around the area.

➤ When your dining buddies won't have anything to do with a vegetarian restaurant, suggest Chinese, Vietnamese, Thai, or Italian. There's always a bunch of vegetarian entrees on the menu.

➤ If there aren't any vegetarian entrees, make up a full meal by selecting a few side dishes. For example, have a baked potato, a house salad, and ask if they'll serve a side of beans. Better yet, request a special vegetarian entree. Most restaurants can be pretty accommodating.

➤ Soup can be a great option in any type of restaurant. Remember to ask if the soup is meat-based or vegetable-based.

➤ Feel free to make substitutions and special requests. For instance, change a bacon, lettuce, and tomato sandwich to a cheese, lettuce, and tomato sandwich, *or* change an order of chicken fajitas to veggie fajitas.

How to Ensure an Adequate Protein Intake

All types of vegetarians can easily meet their protein needs. Protein does not discriminate, it's found in both animal and plant foods. Low-fat dairy and eggs can provide generous amounts of protein for vegetarians that will dare to eat them, and for the "that's absolutely out of the question" vegans, become close pals with tofu, nuts, seeds, lentils, and tempeh. Also, flip back to Chapter 3 and refresh your memory on complementary proteins, that is, making a complete protein (a protein containing all of the essential amino acids) by combining two or more incomplete plant proteins.

The Many Faces of Soy Protein

Decades ago, soy foods were one of the world's best kept secrets. Now, finally out of the closet and raring to jump into just about any of your recipes, soy protein can boost protein, calcium, and the iron content of almost any dish. Go ahead and experiment by incorporating some of the following varieties into your meals, and remember that unflavored soy will take on any flavor you cook or marinate with.

Soymilk   Start your day with a glass of soymilk, or pour it over your cereal for breakfast. Soymilk provides about 4–10 grams of protein per one cup serving, and can be found in low-fat and flavored varieties.

Isolated Soy Protein   This powdery substance is literally 90% pure protein since most of the fat and carbohydrate have been discarded. It's made from defatted soy flour and can be strategically blended into muffins, pancakes, and cookies to help boost your daily protein. A 1-ounce serving (approx 4 TBS.) contains between 13–23 grams of protein.

Soy Flour   Another great way to hike up the protein in your baked products. Soy flour can be used for quick breads, muffins, cookies, and brownies, and $^1/_2$ cup serving supplies 22 grams of protein.

Textured Soy Protein (TSP), also called Textured Vegetable Protein (TVP)   This is made from defatted soy flour, and takes on a granular, flake, or chunk characteristic. TSP comes both plain and flavored, and can be mixed into chili, tacos, veggie burgers, vegetarian casseroles, and stews. When mixed with water, 1 cup prepared provides 22 grams of protein.

Vegetable-Type Soybeans   These dry mature soybeans are loaded with 14 grams of protein per $^{1}/_{2}$ cup serving. What's more, they also contain fiber—double bonus. Tasting both sweet and buttery, their flavor makes them a nice addition to stir-fry dishes, salads, and soups.

Resources
Although tofu and other soy proteins contain some fat, it's very low in saturated fat and contains no cholesterol.

For more information and free brochures on soy protein call 1-800-TALK-SOY.

Tempeh   This cultured soyfood has a tender, chewy consistency that makes it a great candidate for grilled sandwiches, chunky soups, salads, casseroles, and chili. A 4-ounce serving provides 17 grams of protein, about 80 milligrams of calcium and 10% of your daily iron.

Tofu   Just about anything goes with this soy protein. "I'll have a tofu a la mode!" It's made from soymilk curds and can be blended, scrambled, stir-fried, grilled, baked—you name it, chances are it can be done with tofu. There are three types of tofu, firm, soft, and silken.

Definition

   Firm Tofu is stiff, dense, and perfect for stir-fry dishes, soups, or anywhere that you want tofu to maintain its shape. A 4-ounce serving of firm tofu supplies 13 grams protein, 120 milligrams calcium, and about 40% of your daily iron.

Soft Tofu provides 9 grams protein, 130 milligrams calcium, and a little less than 40% of your daily iron from a 4-ounce serving. Soft tofu is good for dishes that require blended tofu (commonly used in soups).

Silken Tofu is creamy and custard-like, and therefore also works well in pureed or blended recipes such as dips, soups, and pies. Silken tofu doesn't provide as much calcium as the more solid tofu varieties (only 40 milligrams), but it is the lowest in fat and is packed with 9 $^{1}/_{2}$ grams of protein per 4-ounce serving.

Ironing Out the Plant Foods

Unfortunately for this less carnivorous crowd, the *heme iron* found in animal foods is much more absorbable than the *nonheme* iron supplied from plants. But that's okay, just go out of your way to eat an abundance of iron-rich plant foods and you'll meet your quota without a hitch. Foods rich in iron include dried beans, spinach, chard, beet greens, blackstrap molasses, bulgur, prune juice, and dried fruits. You may also find that your favorite breakfast cereals are fortified with this mineral. Another trick of the trade is to boost the amount of iron absorbed at a meal by including a food rich in vitamin C (tomatoes, orange juice, and so on). For further information on increasing iron see Chapter 8.

Searching for Non-Dairy Calcium

For the lacto and ovolactos, the low-fat dairy is brimming with calcium. On the other hand, for all you vegans it's definitely going to take some planning; but you too can meet your daily calcium requirements by including collard greens, broccoli, kale, turnip greens, calcium-fortified orange juice, calcium-fortified grains, and like your American Express, *never* leave home without your calcium-fortified soymilk products (including tofu, soybeans, and tempeh).

Have You Had Enough B-12 Today?

Getting enough of the vitamin B-12 can also be somewhat of an obstacle for strict vegans, simply because B-12 is primarily from animal-derived foods. Once again, you lactos and ovolactos are off the hook since the dairy and eggs provide enough to satisfy your daily requirements. However, when it comes to the vegan gang, you gotta dig a little deeper. Try to buy food products that are B-12 fortified such as cereals, breads, *some* soy-analogs, and possibly tempeh. You may also want to pop a B-12 supplement providing 100% of the RDA, just to be on the safe side.

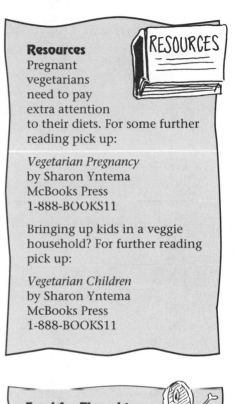

Resources
Pregnant vegetarians need to pay extra attention to their diets. For some further reading pick up:

Vegetarian Pregnancy by Sharon Yntema McBooks Press 1-888-BOOKS11

Bringing up kids in a veggie household? For further reading pick up:

Vegetarian Children by Sharon Yntema McBooks Press 1-888-BOOKS11

Food for Thought
Vegans who don't eat dairy, and aren't regularly out in the sun, should buy foods fortified with vitamin D, *or* speak with their doctor about vitamin D supplemetation.

Don't Forget the Kitchen Zinc

Not only do you have to get all of the necessary RDA of calcium, protein, B-12, and other nutrients, yet another concern for the strict vegetarian is getting a fair share of zinc. Although this mineral is found in whole-grain products, tofu, nuts, seeds, and wheat germ, our bodies absorb much less "plant zinc" than "animal zinc." Therefore, vegetarians need to pay particular attention to getting an abundance of this mineral.

MENU **Ready Made Menu**

A day in the life of a vegan.

Menu 1

Breakfast
Amaranth Flakes with soy milk
Fresh blueberries and raspberries
English muffin topped with peach preserves

Lunch
Peanut butter and banana sandwich
Cup of vegetarian chili topped with scallions
Glass of low-fat soymilk

Snack
Mixture of dried fruit and walnuts
Glass of juice or soymilk

Dinner
Vegetable-tempeh stir-fry (carrots, broccoli,
cauliflower, and tempeh) with brown rice
Sweet potato
Steamed kale sprinkled with sesame seeds
Glass of soymilk

Dessert
Rice Dream (ice cream substitute)
Sliced bananas

Menu 2

Breakfast
Scrambled tofu (see recipe) with whole wheat toast
Bowl of oatmeal with chopped dates and almonds
Glass of cranberry-orange juice

Lunch
Bowl of lentil soup with sourdough rolls
Carrot sticks with hummus dip
Glass of juice or soymilk

Snack
Piece of banana bread
Glass of soymilk

Dinner
Whole wheat tortilla stuffed with beans, salsa,
and arugula
Spinach salad drizzled with olive oil and red
wine vinegar

Dessert
Baked apple with maple syrup and chopped
walnuts

Resources

Order some of these *award winning* vegetarian cookbooks:

Skinny Vegetarian Entrees
by Phyllis Magida and
 Sue Spliter
Surrey Books
1-800-326-4430

New Vegetarian Cuisine
by Linda Rosensweig, from
 the pages of *Prevention
 Magazine*
Rosedale Books
1-800-848-4735

The Enchanted Broccoli Forest
by Mollie Katzen
Ten Speed Press
1-800-841-2665

Simply Vegan—2nd Edition
by Debra Wasserman

The Vegetarian Times Cookbook
Macmillan Publishers
1-800-428-5331

The Vegetarian Resource Group
1-410-366-8343

Remarkably "Meatless" Recipes

Cajun Red Beans and Rice

Serves four

1 cup long grain white rice	2 cups water
1 15 ¹/₄ oz. can kidney beans, drain and rinse	2 tsp. paprika
1 cup canned, crushed tomatoes	1 tsp. Worcestershire
¹/₂ onion, peel and dice ¹/₄ inch	pinch cayenne pepper
1 green bell pepper, dice ¹/₄ inch	¹/₄ tsp. garlic powder
2 bay leaves	4 TBS. chopped green onion

Place all ingredients (except for the chopped, green onions) in a large sauce pan, cover and bring to a boil. Reduce to a simmer and cook 15–20 minutes until rice is tender and liquid is evaporated. Top each portion with 1 TBS. of chopped green onion. Balance out this meal with a dark, leafy green salad tossed with nonfat Italian salad dressing.

Nutrient Analysis for One Serving

Calories 290, Total Fat 1 gram

Saturated Fat 0 grams, Fiber 7 grams

Protein 10 grams, Sodium 170 mg, Cholesterol 0 mg

Copyright by *Food for Health Newsletter*, 1996. Reprinted with their permission.

Vegetarian Spinach Lasagna

Serves eight

2 lbs. low-fat ricotta cheese

4 cups skim milk mozzarella cheese, shredded

1 32 oz. jar of tomato/marinara sauce (low-sodium)

1 package lasagna noodles, uncooked

2 10-12 oz. boxes of frozen spinach, chopped

$^1/_2$ TBS. oregano

1 whole egg + 2 egg whites

$^3/_4$ tsp. pepper

garlic and basil to taste

non-stick cooking spray

1 cup water (for cooking only)

Cook and drain spinach well, then set aside. Mix together ricotta cheese, eggs, pepper, garlic, oregano, basil, and only half of the mozzarella cheese. Add in spinach and mix again thoroughly. Coat lasagna pan with non-stick spray and preheat oven to 350°. Cover the bottom of pan with tomato sauce and then place down a layer of the uncooked lasagna noodles. Next, spread $^1/_2$ of the spinach-cheese mixture evenly on top...and repeat the layers (noodles and then the remaining spinach-cheese mixture). Place on top one more layer of noodles (total of 3 noodle layers) and pour on the remaining tomato sauce. Sprinkle on the other half of the mozzarella cheese. Last, pour the water around the edge of the pan (this will cook the noodles) and cover tightly with tin foil. Bake for 1 hour and 15 minutes, until bubbling. Let stand and cool for 15 minutes before slicing.

Nutrient Analysis for One Serving

Calories 243, Total Fat 7.5 grams

Saturated Fat 3 grams, Fiber 3 grams

Protein 19 grams, Sodium 479 mg, Cholesterol 43 mg

*From the kitchen of Ellen Schloss

Chunky Vegetarian Chili

Serves six

$^1/_2$ cup texturized vegetable protein (TVP)

$^1/_4$ cup boiling water

$^1/_2$ TBS. olive oil

1 large onion, diced

3 cloves garlic, minced

2 medium carrots, chopped

2 medium celery stalks, chopped

1 green bell pepper, seeded and chopped

8 ounces mushrooms, quartered

juice of one lemon

$^1/_2$ tsp. dried basil

$^1/_2$ tsp. dried oregano

¹/₈ tsp. red pepper flakes	1 15-ounce can kidney beans
1 ¹/₂ tsp. chili powder	1 28-ounce can crushed tomatoes
1 ¹/₂ tsp. ground cumin	1 TBS. tomato paste
1 large tomato, chopped	¹/₂ TBS. Marsala wine (optional)
1 15-ounce can pinto beans	2–4 TBS. fresh chives and/or parsley (optional)

Combine the TVP and boiling water in a bowl and set aside. Meanwhile, heat oil in a large stock pot, add onions and sauté until soft (about 3 minutes). Next, add garlic, carrots, celery, pepper, mushrooms, lemon juice, and spices. Cook over medium heat covered for 5 minutes.

Stir in TVP, beans, chopped tomato, and crushed tomatoes. Bring to a simmer. Cook uncovered over low heat for 15 minutes, stirring occasionally. Add Marsala wine and tomato paste, and simmer again for an additional 5 minutes. Remove pot from heat and stir in fresh herbs. Ladle the chili into bowls and garnish with a dollop of low-fat sour cream and chopped red onion. Serve with a fresh loaf of whole-grain bread.

Nutrient Analysis for One Serving (chili only)

Calories 330, Total Fat 2.4 grams

Saturated Fat 0 grams, Fiber 14 grams

Protein 22 grams Sodium 400 mg, Cholesterol 0 mg

*From the kitchen of Meredith Gunsberg

Scrambled Tofu

Serves four

16 ounces of firm tofu	dash of ground cumin
5 TBS. of water	dash of garlic powder
2 TBS. mellow barley light miso	fresh ground pepper to taste

¹/₂ tsp. tumeric

Mash tofu in a small saucepan. In a separate bowl, whisk together all remaining ingredients. Heat tofu over medium flame, and immediately add in the miso mixture. Stir constantly until the scrambled tofu mixture is heated through. Serve hot with toast and ketchup if desired.

Nutrient Analysis for One Serving (tofu only)

Calories 82, Total Fat 4 grams

Saturated Fat 1 gram, Fiber 0 grams

Protein 8 grams, Sodium 32 mg, Cholesterol 0 mg

*From the kitchen of Meredith Gunsberg

Cucumber Yogurt Dip

Serves four

1 large cucumber, peeled, seeded, and grated   2 cloves garlic, pressed

1 cup nonfat plain yogurt   juice of one small lemon

1 TBS. fresh dill, chopped fine   1–2 tsp. fresh chives, chopped fine

Combine all ingredients (except chives and dill), and mix thoroughly. Sprinkle chives on top before serving. Serve with pita bread and plenty of raw vegetables. Yields just over 1 cup.

Nutrient Analysis for One Serving ($1/4$ of dip)

Calories 32, Total Fat 0 grams

Saturated Fat 0 grams, Fiber 0 grams

Protein 3 grams, Sodium 270 mg, Cholesterol 0 mg

*From the kitchen of Meredith Gunsberg

The Least You Need to Know

➤ *Vegans* are the strictest and avoid all meats, dairy, and eggs. *Lacto-vegetarians* eat dairy, but avoid all meat and eggs. *Ovolacto-vegetarians* eat dairy and eggs, but avoid all meat.

➤ Vegetarians (especially vegans) need to be extra responsible about getting enough protein, calcium, vitamin D, vitamin B-12, iron, and zinc.

➤ Lots of non-animal foods provide protein. Nuts, seeds, legumes, and soy-based products are all great sources. The less strict lactos and ovolactos can also obtain protein from dairy products and eggs. The key for the vegetarian is to eat plenty of complementary proteins to get all that are required.

➤ Soy protein can help boost the protein, calcium, and iron content of most any meal.

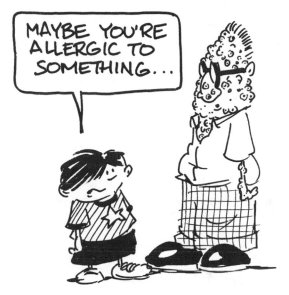

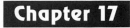

Chapter 17

Food Allergies and Other Ailments

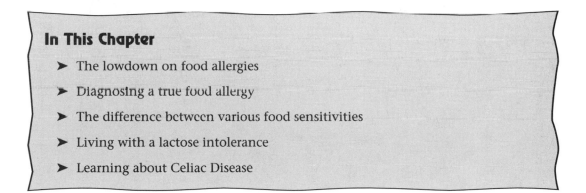

In This Chapter

➤ The lowdown on food allergies

➤ Diagnosing a true food allergy

➤ The difference between various food sensitivities

➤ Living with a lactose intolerance

➤ Learning about Celiac Disease

Do you break out in hives from the mere mention of a peanut? Do you bolt for the bathroom after ingesting anything made with milk? Does the smell of seafood cause your stomach to churn? Hey, even my own grandma, Mary, sneezes repeatedly after devouring her favorite ice cream.

For millions of Americans, symptoms like these can turn the pleasurable act of eating into an uncomfortable and sometimes dangerous situation. In fact, it's estimated that two out of five American adults claim to have *some* type of food sensitivity, ranging from severe food allergies, to less serious (but often equally bothersome) food intolerances. This chapter provides an inside look at the variety of food hypersensitivities, and finally sorts through the confusion, controversy, and skepticism regarding what's what in the world of tasty offenders.

Understanding Food Allergies

Food for Thought
The word "allergy" comes from the Greek words *allos* meaning other, and *ergon* meaning working. In other words, the immune system is working other than normally expected.

Food for Thought
Some people are diagnosed with allergies to food additives such as sulfites (food preservatives), tartrazine (food colorings), and MSG (flavor enhancer), and therefore must check ingredient labels with extreme care and ask lots of questions when dining out.

A true *food allergy* is a hypersensitive reaction that occurs when your immune system responds abnormally to harmless proteins that are found in food. That is, your body misinterprets something good as an intruder and produces antibodies to "halt" the invasion. Sort of like *every* episode of *Three's Company*. Remember the time Jack snuck in late one night, and Chrissy and Janet mistook him for a robber and clobbered him over the head? It's pretty much the same thing with food allergies, only in this case you can't just laugh and shut off the TV; you actually experience the miserable symptoms firsthand.

The most common food culprits linked to allergic reactions are wheat, shellfish, nuts, soybeans, corn, the protein in cow's milk, and eggs. Furthermore, the organs most commonly affected are the skin (symptoms include skin rashes, hives, itching, and swelling), the respiratory tract (symptoms include difficulty breathing and "hay fever"), and the gastrointestinal tract (symptoms include nausea, bloating, diarrhea, and vomiting). Some allergic reactions are so severe they can even provoke anaphylactic shock, a life-threatening, whole-body response, which requires immediate medical attention.

Definition

Food sensitivity is a general term used to describe *any* abnormal response to food or food additive.

Food allergy is an over reaction by the body's immune system, usually triggered by protein-containing foods (such as cow's milk, nuts, soybeans, shellfish, eggs, and wheat).

Anaphylactic shock is a life-threatening, whole-body allergic reaction to an offending substance. Symptoms include, swelling of the mouth and throat, difficulty breathing, drop in blood pressure, and loss of consciousness. In other words, get help fast!

Food intolerance is an adverse reactions to foods that generally do *not* involve the immune system (such as lactose intolerance).

Food poisoning is an adverse reaction caused by contaminated food (micro-organisms, parasites, or other toxins).

Antibodies are large protein molecules that are produced by the body's immune system in response to foreign substances.

Diagnosing a True Food Allergy

Many folks view this whole food sensitivity business as faddism and quackery, and unfortunately we have earned this mindset! Did you know that out of the gazillions of people that think they have a food allergy, less than 2 percent of the American adult population actually have one? So why does the idea of a food allergy get so recklessly thrown around? One reason may be because people are often quick to blame physical ailments on food. Maybe you read some bogus article and thought, "Yeah that sounds like me, I guess I have a food allergy." Another *aggravating* reason for all the misdiagnosis are those so-called "allergy quacks" that grab your hard earned money and diagnose you with the "allergy flavor of the month." And ever get a load of some of the quick remedies they suggest: mix $^2/_3$ bottle lemongrass with $^1/_3$ bottle of ginseng. Drink it while doing a one-armed handstand!

In today's world, a true food allergy can be properly diagnosed with scientifically sound methods of testing. If you think you may be suffering from an allergic response to certain food substances get it checked out. The first step is to find a qualified and reputable physician who has been certified by the American Board of Allergy and Immunology. Ask your primary doctor for a referral, *or* call the American Academy of Allergy and Immunology at 1-800-822-2762, and they'll set you up with a physician in your area. Next, schedule an appointment. Here's what you can expect:

Food for Thought
Some people have such severe food allergies that they can even exhibit symptoms from the following:

➤ By kissing the lips of someone who has eaten the offending food

➤ By just smelling and inhaling the offending food while it cooks

➤ Coming into contact with utensils that have touched the offending food

Food for Thought
Statistics report up to 7% of all infants and small children are allergic to certain foods, a much higher incidence than among American adults (less than 2%).

➤ **Thorough Medical History**   A detailed history of both you and your family's medical background will be taken. Special attention will be given to the type and frequency of your symptoms, along with when the symptoms occur in relation to eating food.

➤ **Complete Physical Examination**   A routine physical exam will be taken with special focus on the areas where you experience the suspected food allergy symptoms.

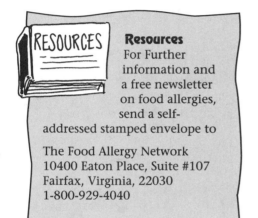

Resources
For Further information and a free newsletter on food allergies, send a self-addressed stamped envelope to

The Food Allergy Network
10400 Eaton Place, Suite #107
Fairfax, Virginia, 22030
1-800-929-4040

Rocky Road
Beware of enthusiasts using "Cytotoxicity tests." These tests involve taking a small sample of blood, then separating out and mixing the white blood cells with specific food extracts to observe for change in shape and size. Because cytotoxicity tests are often unreliable, they should not be used for diagnosing food allergies and are not recommended by the American Academy of Allergy and Immunology.

➤ **Food Elimination Diets**   The doctor will probably have you keep a food diary while you eliminate *all* suspicious foods from your diet. The allergist may then tell you to slowly, *one at a time,* add back these foods to your diet so that you can specifically identify which foods may cause an adverse reaction.

➤ **Skin Tests**   An extract of a particular food is placed on the skin (usually arm or back) and then pricked or scratched into the skin to look for a reaction of itching or swelling. Not 100% reliable since some people that are not necessarily food allergic do develop skin rashes. On the other hand, some people do not show skin reactions, but do indeed have true allergic responses when the foods are eaten.

➤ **RAST Tests (Radioallergosorbent tests)**   This test involves mixing small samples of your blood with food extracts in a test tube. If you are truly allergic to a particular food, your blood will produce antibodies to fight off the food extract it has been mixed with. This type of test has the advantage of being performed outside your body and therefore you don't have to deal with the discomfort of itching and swelling if it proves to be positive. Note: This test will only foretell of an allergy, not the extent of sensitivity to the offending food.

➤ **Double-Blind Food Challenge Tests**   This type of test must be performed under close supervision, preferably in an allergist's office or hospital and is considered the "gold standard" in food allergy testing. Two capsules of dried food are prepared, one with the real McCoy and another with a nonreactive substance. Neither doctor nor patient knows which one is which (a double blind challenge). These challenges can rule out, as well as detect, allergies or intolerances to foods and other food substances such as additives.

Treating a True Food Allergy

So what's the treatment once you're diagnosed with a true food allergy? Avoid anything with the offending food!

Although this list is *not* a substitute for consulting with a registered dietitian, it can provide a pretty good idea of which food ingredients should be avoided after you've been diagnosed with one of the following food allergies:

Cow's milk   Check labels very carefully and avoid all foods with the following ingredients: milk, yogurt, cheese, cottage cheese, custard, casein, whey, ghee, milk solids, curds, sodium caseinate, lactoglobulin, lactalbumin, milk chocolate, buttermilk, cream, sour cream, and butter.

Wheat   Avoid all foods with the following ingredients: wheat, wheat germ, all-purpose flour, duram flour, cracker meal, couscous, bulgur, whole wheat berries, cake flour, gluten flour, pastry flour, graham flour, semolina, bran, cereal or malt extract, modified food starch, farina, and graham.

Corn   Avoid all foods with the following ingredients: fresh, canned, or frozen corn (regular and creamed versions); hominy; corn grits; maize; cornmeal; corn flour; corn sugar; baking powder; corn syrup; cornstarch; modified food starch; dextrin; malto-dextrins; dextrose; fructose; lactic acid; corn alcohol; vegetable gums; sorbitol; vinegar; and popcorn. Some good news is that studies show most allergic individuals can safely eat *pure corn oil,* since it does not contain the protein found in corn.

Soy   Avoid all foods with the following ingredients: soy, lecithin, tofu, textured vegetable protein (TVP), tempeh, modified food starch, soy miso, soy sauce, teriyaki sauce, and soybean flour.

Nuts   Folks that are allergic to peanuts and other types of nuts not only need to avoid the obvious plain nuts and nut butters, but also need to be on the look out for "hidden" nuts that are tossed into baked goods, vegetarian dishes, candies, cereals, salads, and chicken stir-fry meals. Good news again, like corn oil, studies show that pure peanut oil is nonallergenic and therefore okay for most folks allergic to nuts.

Eggs   Avoid all foods that indicate the presence of an egg by listing any of the following ingredients: powdered or dry egg, egg white, dried egg yolk, egg substitute, eggnog, albumin, ovalbumin, ovomucin, ovomucoid, vitellin, ovovitellin, livetin, globulin, and ovoglobulin egg albumin.

Shellfish   Avoid all shrimp, lobster, prawn, crab, crawfish, crayfish, clams, oysters, scallops, snails, octopus, squid, mussels, and geoducks.

So What's the Difference Between a Food Allergy and Food Intolerance?

Simple, the difference lies in how your body handles the offending food. Where a food allergy affects the body's immune system, a food intolerance generally affects the body's metabolism. In other words, the body cannot properly digest a food or food substance, resulting in "intestinal chaos," alias the gurgles.

What's a Lactose Intolerance All About?

Food for Thought
Don't confuse a lactose intolerance with a milk allergy. Where a lactose intolerance involves difficulty digesting the milk sugar lactose, a milk allergy involves an allergic reaction from the protein components in cow's milk. What's more, folks who suffer from milk allergies cannot even tolerate any of the reduced-lactose specialty products because the part of the milk they are allergic to (milk proteins) is still present.

If you can't stomach milk, and experience bloating, nausea, cramping, excessive gas, *or* a bad case of the runs after eating a dairy food, you are not alone! In fact, it's estimated that 30 to 50 million Americans suffer from some degree of a lactose intolerance, which is the inability to digest the milk sugar *lactose*. In fact, I once had a client who told me that he visited so many men's rooms while touring through Europe he was ready to write *The Complete Idiot's Guide to European Bathrooms*.

So why can't some people tolerate dairy foods? People who are lactose intolerant are unable to produce enough of the enzyme *lactase*, which is responsible for the digestion of lactose in your gut. Just imagine trying to tear down a skyscraper without a bulldozer, it's just not gonna happen! Just like the bulldozer, lactose is dependent on *lactase* to be broken down, digested, and absorbed in the bloodstream. What's more, this type of intolerance affects people at different levels. Where one person may dash for the bathroom after just one sip of milk, others can tolerate small amounts of dairy without any problem.

Who Generally Tends to Have a Problem Digesting Milk?

➤ Up to 70 percent of the entire world's population does not produce enough of the enzyme lactase, and therefore has some degree of lactose intolerance.

➤ In the United States alone, the following groups experience some or all symptoms of lactose intolerance

Over 80% of Asian Americans

79% of Native Americans

75% of African Americans

51% Hispanic Americans

21% Caucasian Americans

➤ In rare cases, some people are born unable to produce the enzyme lactase due to a congenital defect.

➤ Following gastric surgery, people taking chronic antibiotics, or anti-inflammatory drugs may also lose their ability (both short-term and long-term) to digest lactose.

➤ People may develop a *temporary* lactose intolerance during a bout of the flu, a stomach virus, or irritable bowel (spastic colon). During these horrid instances, your doctor will probably tell you to avoid all milk and dairy since the enzyme lactase is easily destroyed with any stomach irritation. In these cases, when you recover, so does your ability to produce lactase.

Living with a Lactose Intolerance

The following are helpful tips for people that have difficulty digesting lactose. As mentioned earlier, the degree of lactose intolerance can vary from person to person, therefore *not* everyone will be able to handle all of the suggestions. Give them each a shot, but be sure that you are in a comfortable place (and as Archie Bunker would say, "have a terlet close by" in case of disaster). Keep in mind that the lactose-containing foods are generally your best sources for the mineral calcium, so children and women with increased calcium requirements should speak with a registered dietitian about ensuring an adequate intake *and* the possibility of calcium supplementation.

➤ Carefully look through the list of food ingredients and check for obvious and *disguised* lactose including, milk, cheese, cream, margarine, sour cream, milk solids, milk chocolate, whey, curds, malted milk, and skim milk solids. Remember that people with severe lactose problems may not be able to tolerate even the small amounts added into pancakes, biscuits, cookies, cakes, instant potatoes, salad dressings, sauces, gravies, lunch meats, soups, powdered coffee creamers, and whipped toppings.

➤ Be aware that a lot of over-the-counter medications have added lactose. Speak with your pharmacist if you're not completely sure what's up.

➤ While most people cannot gulp down a straight glass of milk, some folks can tolerate smaller amounts of dairy combined with other foods. For instance, try a bowl of cereal with fruit and *milk*, or a slice of pizza with lots of veggies (easy on the *cheese)*, or a ham sandwich with one slice of *cheese*.

➤ Some people with L.I. can tolerate yogurt because the bacteria in the yogurt actually metabolizes the milk sugar lactose for you.

➤ Also try cultured buttermilk and sweet acidophilis milk. Some folks find them easier to digest than the regular milk.

➤ When real ice cream is a lethal poison, try a non-dairy substitute like Toffuti™ or Rice Dream™.

➤ Stock up on special lactose-reduced products including lactaid milk, Dairy Ease™, lactaid cottage cheese, and lactaid ice cream.

➤ Try the special tablets and drops that you can add into regular milk; they will almost completely breakdown the lactose after sitting for about 24 hours in the fridge.

➤ Also look for special lactase enzyme pills in your pharmacy that you can swallow *before* eating or drinking a dairy product. This comes in handy when you think you may be thrown into a "hairy-dairy" situation.

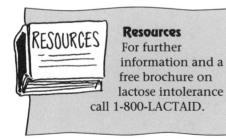

Resources
For further information and a free brochure on lactose intolerance call 1-800-LACTAID.

➤ In severe cases, even the lactose-reduced products may not be tolerated. But don't cheat your body of calcium just because you can't stomach the dairy. Buy calcium-fortified juice, calcium-fortified soymilk, and any other calcium-fortified food products you can get your hands on. *P.S.:* Definitely speak with your physician or a registered dietitian about calcium supplementation.

Resources

The Candida Connection

This theory speculates that some people are hypersensitive to a yeast fungus called *candida*. People advocating this theory claim that candida can multiply, weaken the immune system, and cause an array of symptoms including everything from headaches to depression. The so-called treatment includes a diet that is void of all yeast, mold-containing foods, fruits, milk, refined carbohydrates (simple sugary carbs), and processed foods.

But before you go eliminating any of your favorite foods from your diet, understand this: Candida *normally* inhabits the mouth, skin, and intestines of healthy people without causing harm or discomfort, therefore this diagnosis is highly unlikely. It's true that some folks do develop real fungal infections on the skin and nails, but there has never been any scientific link connecting candida to the other suggested ailments, *or* that the avoidance of certain foods can lessen the yeast formation in your body.

Celiac Disease: Life without Wheat, Rye, Barley, and Oats

Another food-related condition (less common than lactose intolerance) is Gluten-Sensitive Enteropathy, better known as celiac disease or gluten intolerance. Celiac disease is a chronic disorder found in genetically susceptible individuals who exhibit severe intestinal distress after eating anything made with *gluten*, a protein found in wheat, rye, barley, and oats. People with this condition must follow a lifelong diet avoiding *all* offending foods, *or* suffer the potential for malnourishment from chronic diarrhea and nutrient malabsorption.

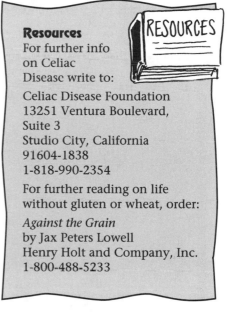

Resources
For further info on Celiac Disease write to:

Celiac Disease Foundation
13251 Ventura Boulevard, Suite 3
Studio City, California 91604-1838
1-818-990-2354

For further reading on life without gluten or wheat, order:

Against the Grain
by Jax Peters Lowell
Henry Holt and Company, Inc.
1-800-488-5233

As you can imagine, life on this diet is no picnic because a bowl of pasta, a plain bagel, cereal, crackers, or even a slice of bread can send a celiac's intestines into a sumo wrestling match. Obviously, with the tremendous amount of food restrictions, members of the Gluten-Free club should consult with a registered dietitian who's extremely knowledgeable in this particular area of nutrition. What's more, become best friends with your local healthfood store, they're celiac-friendly and generally carry the specialty items you'll need for your daily diet.

Irritable Bowel Syndrome

Although not completely understood, Irritable Bowel Syndrome (IBS) seems to be more common these days than the sniffles. With symptoms ranging from excessive gas, cramping, bloating, and intermittent bouts of constipation and diarrhea, IBS (also called a spastic colon) usually has *nothing* to do with food allergies or intolerances. Instead, it is more likely a functional problem with the muscular movement of your intestines. In fact, it's generally diagnosed when all of the serious gastrointestinal ailments are ruled out.

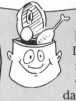

Food for Thought
Despite the widespread notion that chocolate, sugar, dairy products, and other fatty foods are responsible for the outbreak of pimples, most dermatologists today *rarely* identify an underlying relationship between acne and diet.

Some doctors say that in certain instances, people can even bring it on with anxiety or nerves.

Dietary treatments that can help alleviate the symptoms include eating slowly, increasing fiber gradually, reducing total fat, drinking lots of water, and regularly exercising. You may also want to keep a food log for a week or two and see if there are any particular foods that exacerbate the symptoms (some common culprits include alcohol, tobacco, caffeine, and spicy foods). Also see if there's a correlation between your work schedule and the days you're feeling bad; some people find that the symptoms *improve* on the weekends when they are relaxing.

The Least You Need to Know

➤ A food allergy is when your body misinterprets a harmless food as an intruder and produces antibodies to fight off the foreign substance.

➤ If you think you may be allergic to a food, get it legitimately checked out with a doctor who is certified by the American Board of Allergy and Immunology.

➤ A food allergy affects the immune system, while a food intolerance generally affects only the digestive system.

➤ Lactose intolerance is the inability to produce enough of the enzyme *lactase,* which is responsible for digesting the milk sugar lactose. Symptoms include bloating, cramping, gas, diarrhea, and nausea.

➤ Celiac Disease is a condition that causes severe malabsorption after ingesting the protein gluten, which is found in wheat, rye, oats, and barley.

➤ Irritable Bowel Syndrome is a functional problem with the muscular movement of the intestines, resulting in intermittent bouts of constipation, diarrhea, bloating, and gas.

Part 5
Nutrition and Fitness For Two

Let the cravings begin! Being pregnant is both exciting and overwhelming, and the importance of good nutrition for mothers-to-be has been stressed over and over again. What's more, today most health experts also encourage exercise, which can help keep moms feeling more fit and mobile during their nine months of growing girth. Read on—in this section I'll provide lots of essential information that will help to manage your—and your child's health.

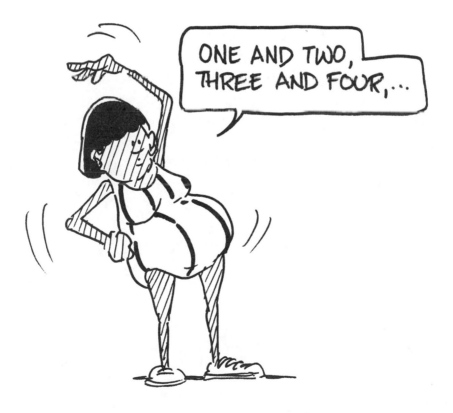

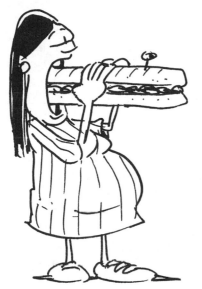

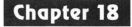

Chapter 18

Feeding Yourself and Your Growing Baby

In This Chapter

➤ Eating for a healthy pregnancy

➤ How much weight should you gain?

➤ Boosting your protein, dairy, iron, and fluid intake

➤ Strategies to reduce constipation, nausea, heartburn, and water retention

Yippee! You're pregnant. Congratulations on your exciting news! This chapter provides all the info you'll need to properly nourish yourself *and* your growing baby. Okay, let the games begin!

Are You Really Eating for Two? Yes and No

Has anyone ever said, "Go ahead and pack it in, you're eating for two people?" Well, that's both true and false. *True* because your food selections will directly affect your growing baby. In other words, eat plenty of quality foods, loaded with nutrients, and you'll shower that growing bambino with all the right ingredients (*or* you eat junk, your baby gets junk!). On the other hand, this statement is also *false* because you're clearly *not* eating for two adults. In fact, your growing baby is only a fraction of your size, so take it easy with those second helpings.

Increased Calories and Protein

It's true that you do need more calories. In fact, during the entire course of your pregnancy you'll need to consume about an extra *80,000 calories*. That's an extra 360 containers of yogurt, *or* 1,800 cups of berries, *or* for all you rebels out there, 2,000 donut holes (don't even think about it!). But obviously this caloric increase is spread out over a nine-month period and only winds up to be approximately 150 extra calories each day during the first trimester (the first three months), and around 350 extra calories each day during the 2nd and 3rd trimesters (the last six months).

You'll also need some extra protein *within* those extra calories because your precious developing fetus needs ample amounts. Getting this increased protein requirement is *not* typically a problem. Most women already overshoot their needs pre-pregnancy, and consuming extra dairy and larger servings of lean meat, fish, poultry, eggs, and legumes will ensure that you're getting enough. For a more detailed description on how much protein you'll need, see the section on adjusting your eating plan later in this chapter.

A Weighty Issue: How Many Pounds Should I Gain?

It seems like the first thing everyone asks about when you return from your doctor's office is *not*, "How did the baby's heartbeat sound?" *Or*, "Did the doctor say anything about the baby's positioning or size?" No, the most commonly asked question is, "How much weight did you gain?" How annoying! It's obvious enough that your belly is growing and that you're visibly gaining weight, but as for the number, it's nobody's business but yours, your doctor, *and of course your mother*! So how many pounds should you gain? Here's what's recommended for most healthy women:

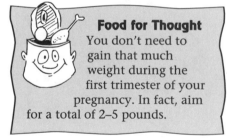

Food for Thought
You don't need to gain that much weight during the first trimester of your pregnancy. In fact, aim for a total of 2–5 pounds.

Pre-pregnancy Weight	Suggested Weight Gain	Weekly Weight Gain For 2nd and 3rd Trimester
Underweight <90% desirable weight	28–40 pounds	>1 pound
Normal Weight (see range in chart) Chapter 22	25–35 pounds	.8–1 pound
Moderately Overweight >120–135% desirable weight	15–25 pounds	.7 pounds
Very Overweight >135% desirable weight	15–20 pounds	.5 pounds

Keep in mind that "desirable" weights fall within a range. You can see where you stand "pre-pregnancy" by comparing your weight in pounds with the chart located in Chapter 22. Also, understand that there are special circumstances where some women will *need* to gain more, some less. For instance, women carrying twins will need to gain about 35–45 pounds, and although women with triplets almost *never* carry full term, (they typically deliver around 33 weeks) if they did, they would need to gain in the vicinity of 50–70 pounds (and hire three full-time nannies and a massage therapist). Rap with your doctor and listen to his or her advice on this weighty issue.

Adjusting Your Eating Plan

Now let's ensure that you're gaining weight with the proper foods. Remember those 5 friendly food groups that have haunted you since page 1? Like the Poltergeist…*They're baa-ack.* Although individual requirements vary depending on calorie needs, the chart below gives some guidance in determining the basics of your diet.

> **Food for Thought**
> Try not to get overly anxious about the weight gain—it's a normal component of a healthy pregnancy. Remember, as long as you eat smart, you'll be back to your old figure in no time!

> **Q and A**
> Where does the extra weight go?
>
> baby: 7–8 pounds
> placenta 1–2 pounds
> amniotic fluid: 1 1/2–2 pounds
> uterine tissue: 2 pounds
> breast tissue: 1–2 pounds
> expanded blood and other fluid volume: 6–10 pounds
> fat: 6–7 pounds
> *Total = 25–35 pounds*

Food Group	Daily Servings	Sample servings
Breads/Grains	6+	1 slice bread, or 1/2 small bagel, or 1 serving cereal, or 1/2 cup cooked rice or pasta
Fruits	3+	1 medium fruit, or 1 cup berries or melon, or 1/2 cup fruit juice
Vegetables	3+	1 cup raw leafy veggies, or 1/2 cup cooked veggies
Dairy	4+	1 cup milk, or 1 cup yogurt, or 3/4 cup cottage cheese, or 1 1/2 ounces of hard cheese

continues

continued

Food Group	Daily Servings	Sample servings
Meat/Poultry/ Fish/Beans/Eggs/ Nuts	2–3	2–3 ounces lean meat, or 2 eggs(limit 2× per week),or $^2/_3$ cup of tofu 2–3 ounces of fish or poultry
Fluids	8+	8 ounces of water, seltzer, and other beverages
Fats/Sweets	moderation	Just try your best to keep these foods to a minimum.

Ready Made Menu

Eating with a "bun in the oven"

Menu #1
Breakfast
cereal with raisins
1 cup low-fat milk
grapefruit juice

Lunch
$^1/_2$ turkey (2 oz.) and
cheese (1 $^1/_2$ oz.)sandwich
vegetable soup (1 cup)
seltzer water

Snack
8 ounces of yogurt and a banana

Dinner
tossed salad with light dressing
chicken breast (5 oz.)
brown rice (1 $^1/_2$ cups)
water

Snack
1 cup low-fat milk
graham crackers

Menu #2
Breakfast
waffles with fresh fruit
1 cup yogurt
glass milk or juice

Lunch
grilled chicken (3 oz.) salad
melba toast or pita
fresh strawberries
water

Snack
pretzels, a peach
1 cup of milk

Dinner
grilled fish (4–5 oz.)
pasta with vegetables, marinara
sauce, and 1 cup broccoli
parmesan cheese
cranberry juice

Snack
frozen yogurt topped with
low-fat granola

Rocky Road

Don't fool yourself into thinking "Hey, I'm pregnant, I can eat *whatever* and *whenever* I want!" Yes, it's true that with pregnancy comes increased caloric and nutrient requirements, but there are ways to meet these needs and there are ways to meet these needs while putting on an extra 20 pounds of flub! I'm not saying that you should deprive yourself of cravings and urges—that's one of the fun things about pregnancy. Just don't cram down fats and sweets from the moment you see the positive sign on the pregnancy test till the time you deliver (*hey I'm pregnant please pass the yodels*). Believe me, that extra weight is *not* all baby. Have you ever heard of a 30–40 pound newborn? The bottom line is that a lot of extra weight gained during your pregnancy is a lot of extra weight you'll be wearing *after* the baby is born.

Why All the Hype on Calcium?

Although this mineral is needed throughout the life cycle it is particularly important during pregnancy. (At last, you finally learn the reason why everyone pesters you to drink milk.) In fact, your daily requirements shoot up from 800 milligrams to 1,200 milligrams when you become pregnant (some experts recommend 1,500 milligrams)—that's approximately 4 servings of dairy (for example, 1 cup of milk + 1 cup pudding + 1 cup fruit yogurt + 1 $\frac{1}{2}$ ounces of hard cheese). As you learned in Chapter 8, calcium is responsible for strong bones and teeth, for the proper functioning of blood vessels, nerves, and muscles, as well as maintaining healthy connective tissue. During pregnancy, calcium is especially critical because you now have to worry about your own bones *and* your growing baby's bones, tissues, and teeth as well. In fact, your baby counts on *your* calcium for normal development, therefore when you skimp on the calcium-rich foods (and don't take supplementation), the calcium in your bones will be supplied to meet the increased demands of the growing fetus. In other words, *hello osteoporosis*. See Chapter 8 for the calcium content of various foods, both dairy and nondairy.

Q and A

Won't the prenatal vitamins cover all the calcium my baby will need?

Definitely not! Prenatal supplements supply about 200–250 milligrams per pill, that's not even one serving from the dairy group.

Food for Thought

Pregnant women with lactose intolerance should eat plenty of *nondairy* calcium-fortified foods, along with the special lactose-reduced products. Also, speak with your physician about calcium supplementation. (For further information on lactose intolerance see Chapter 17.)

Hiking Up the Iron

Ever wonder why the prenatal vitamins are loaded with iron? It's because during pregnancy your body requires about double the amount of this mineral than usual. In fact, you go from normally needing 15 milligrams (remember the RDA?), to requiring a daily dose of 30 milligrams when you're expecting. So *why* exactly do pregnant women require more iron? Remember, iron is found in your blood, and is responsible for carrying and delivering oxygen to every cell in your body. Being that pregnant women have an *expanded* blood volume, it makes sense that more blood requires more iron. Also, think about having to supply both your cells with oxygen, *and* the cells of your growing baby. Once again, this greater demand for oxygen requires greater amounts of the "O2 delivery boy," iron.

Food for Thought

Because nursing your baby *also* requires an increase in calories, protein, calcium, and a variety of other nutrients, nursing women will also benefit from following the same general eating guidelines discussed in this chapter. Notice how the demands for calories, protein, calcium, folic acid, and iron increase during pregnancy and lactation.

	Pre-preg.	Pregnant	Lactating/Breast Feeding
Calories		+300	+500
Protein (gr)	44–50	60	59–65 (first six mos.) 56–62 (second six mos.)
Calcium (mg)	800	1,200–1,500	1,200
Folic Acid (mg)	200	400	300
Iron (mg)	15	30	15

And just because the prenatal vitamins are brimming with the stuff, don't think you can slack off in the food department. Understand that prenatal supplements (providing around 30–60 milligrams) are merely the "just in case" backup—you'll still need to pay particular attention to eating lots of iron-rich foods. Notice on the eating plan that you require 2–3 servings of protein foods each day? This will help satisfy your body's extra demand for *both* protein and the mineral iron because the best absorbable iron is found in the foods within this group. For further tips on boosting your iron flip back to Chapter 8.

Best sources—heme-iron:
animal foods such as beef, pork, lamb, veal, chicken, turkey, fish, seafood, and eggs.

Good sources—nonheme-iron:
non-animal foods such as enriched breads and cereals, beans, dried fruits, seeds, nuts, broccoli, spinach, collard greens, and blackstrap molasses.

> **Food for Thought**
> Sometimes the increased iron can cause constipation, diarrhea, dark colored stools, and abdominal discomfort. Don't be alarmed, it's just par for the course. Be sure to increase your fiber and fluids and move around as much as possible!

> **Food for Thought**
> Pregnant women have increased needs for calories, protein, calcium, iron, folic acid, zinc, vitamin C, and several other B-vitamins including B-1, B-2, B-3, B-6, and B-12.

Keep on Drinkin', Sippin', Gulpin', and Guzzlin'!

Proper hydration is another vital component for a healthy pregnancy. Did you know that the average female is about 55–65% water, and the average newborn is about 85% water? During this 9-month period of bodily change, shift, and growth (and boy do I mean change, shift, and growth), your fluid demands skyrocket for the following reasons:

➤ You now need to maintain your *expanded* blood supply and fluid volume. You see, through the blood and lymphatic system, water helps deliver oxygen and other nutrients all over your body.

➤ Like always, fluids are needed to help wash down your food and assist in nutrient absorption.

➤ Extra fluids, along with fiber, can help to alleviate some of the bothersome plumbing problems, alias "mom to be" constipation.

> **Way to Go**
> "Favorable Fluids" you should be guzzling down are: water, club soda, bottled water, vegetable juice, seltzer, fruit juice, and low-fat milk.
>
> Liquids you should steer clear of are: alcohol, coffee, tea, soft drinks, diet cola (and other artificially sweetened drinks), and herbal teas.

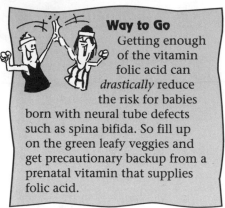

Way to Go

Getting enough of the vitamin folic acid can *drastically* reduce the risk for babies born with neural tube defects such as spina bifida. So fill up on the green leafy veggies and get precautionary backup from a prenatal vitamin that supplies folic acid.

➤ Fluid provides a cushion for the developing fetus and also helps to lubricate all of your joints.

➤ Lastly, fluid is needed for the normal functioning of *every* cell in your body.

Are you convinced yet? Good. Also realize that in some pregnant instances you may need even *more* than the already increased amount. For example, if you're perspiring in hot weather, *or* when you're exercising, *or* if you have any type of fever, vomiting, or diarrhea (obviously in the latter case contact your doctor immediately).

Foods to Forget!

The following is a suggested list of foods to *avoid* until after the baby is born.

Raw foods   Because these foods can increase your risk for bacterial infection, avoid anything raw including sushi and other seafood, beef tartar, undercooked poultry, raw or unpasteurized milk, soft cooked and poached eggs, or raw egg that's possibly found in eggnog, cookie dough, caesar salads, and milkshakes.

Nitrates, Nitrites, and Nitrosamines   These are possible cancer-causing chemicals and are found in hot dogs, bacon, bologna, and other processed cold cuts.

Alcohol   Since alcohol can damage the developing fetus (Fetal Alcohol Syndrome), avoid all beer, wine, and liquor.

Caffeine   Although there is insufficient evidence to conclude that caffeine adversely affects reproduction in humans, it does cross through the placenta and into the baby's body. Therefore it is smart to avoid coffee, tea, and other highly caffeinated beverages.

Herbal teas   Some herbal teas can have medicinal properties. Check out anything questionable with your nutritionist or physician before assuming that it's okay to drink.

MSG   Monosodium glutamate can cause uncomfortable side effects for the pregnant mom including headaches, dizziness, and nausea.

Artificial sweeteners   This is a tough judgment call. While some health professionals claim artificial sweeteners are perfectly safe during pregnancy, others say you should completely avoid them. In my opinion, why play around with your baby's health—get rid of them for a brief nine months.

Q and A

What is gestational diabetes?

Gestational diabetes is the onset of high blood sugar (or carbohydrate intolerance) that is generally detected around the 28th week of pregnancy. Because this condition is caused by the placenta putting out large doses of anti-insulin hormones, as soon as the placenta is removed (during the baby's delivery), the condition disappears in almost all cases. People who are diagnosed with gestational diabetes have very specific dietary concerns and should work with a qualified nutritionist (registered dietitian) on appropriate meal planning.

Way to Go!

Dig in and blast your baby with vitamins!

Fruits rich in Vitamin C:
orange, grapefruit, mango, strawberries, papaya, raspberries, tangerine, kiwi, cantaloupe, guava, lemon, orange juice, grapefruit juice, and other vitamin C-fortified juices.

Vegetables rich in Vitamin C:
broccoli, tomato, sweet potato, pepper, kale, cabbage, Brussels sprouts, rutabaga, cauliflower, and spinach.

Fruits rich in Vitamin A:
apricot, cantaloupe, papaya, mango, prunes, peach, nectarine, tangerine, watermelon, and guava.

Vegetables rich in Vitamin A:
broccoli, Brussels sprouts, carrots, collard greens, escarole, dark green lettuce, spinach, sweet potato, kale, butternut squash, chicory, red pepper, and tomato juice.

The Many Trials and Tribulations of Having a Baby

While embarking on the beginnings of motherly bliss, some women glow and others, shall I say, turn green. I was one of the unlucky green women (actually, my husband described it more like a interesting shade of grayish blue). Although agonizing and uncomfortable (*to put it mildly*), these lousy side effects including constipation, nausea, water retention, and heartburn, are merely normal "pregnancy" occurrences and most certainly worth the beautiful end product.

The "Uh-Oh, Better Get Drano" Feeling

Most pregnant women experience the constipation blues at one time or another during the nine-month haul. So why does food tend to stop dead in it's tracks before reaching its final destination anyway? Unfortunately, there are a bunch of explanations.

➤ Hormonal changes

➤ The increased pressure on your intestinal tract as your baby grows in size

➤ All of the extra iron in your prenatal supplements

➤ Not enough fiber in your diet

➤ Not drinking enough fluids

➤ The plain old lack of exercise

Yes, it's true that the first three circumstances are completely uncontrollable, but let's focus on the last three: fiber, fluid, and exercise, which are quite controllable and can *dramatically* decrease your plumbing problems!

First, increase your dietary fiber by eating more fresh fruit, veggies, and whole grain foods. Better yet, flip back to the fiber chapter (Chapter 6) and read the tips for boosting your daily intake. Next, drink a ton of fluids. And lastly, stay tuned for Chapter 19, which explains how to "Move and Groove with a Bun in the Oven." That is, incorporate a safe and effective exercise plan (with your doc's okay of course) into your pregnant schedule.

UGH! That Nagging Nausea!

Commonly known as "morning sickness," this awful nausea and vomiting can occur at *any* time of the day, so don't be misled. One bit of reassuring news: Although horridly unpleasant, it's *normal* and thought to simply be a side effect from the hormonal changes that take place during pregnancy. What's more, if you've become best friends with your bathroom (or any and every bathroom you may be near), hang in there (*literally*), the nausea usually disappears by week 14.

Here are some tips to help reduce the nausea:

➤ Nibble on carbohydrate-rich foods throughout the day. They are easy to digest and will provide your body with some energy (calories). For example, bagels, pretzels, crackers, cereal, and rice cakes are all primo snacks.

➤ If you tend to be nauseated in the early morning, keep some of the above carbs by your bed. Pop something into your mouth *before* getting up, this will start the digestive process and get rid of excess stomach acid.

➤ Most women find cold foods easier to tolerate than hot foods; however, everyone is unique. What makes one woman sick may be soothing to another. In other words, listen to your own body and go ahead with whatever works best for you.

➤ Avoid any sharp cooking odors, and open the windows for some fresh air.

➤ When solid foods are just *not* going to happen, suck on an ice pop, frozen fruit bars, or sip on lemonade and fruit juice.

➤ Avoid high-fat foods since they sit longer in your stomach and can exacerbate the nausea.

➤ Sometimes iron supplements can intensify nausea. If you are taking iron pills, try taking them with a snack or two hours after a meal with some ginger-ale. If the nausea persists, you may also want to speak with your doctor about possibly holding off on the iron until you feel better.

➤ Do *not* take prenatal vitamins on an empty stomach—take them with a meal or snack.

Contact your doctor immediately if you have persistent vomiting, are losing weight, or are too nauseated to take in fluids.

What's All the Swelling About?

Edema is the uncomfortable swelling, or retention of water that occurs primarily in your feet, ankles, and hands during pregnancy. As long as there's no increase in blood pressure or protein in the urine, edema is normal and unfortunately tends to get worse in the last trimester (your last 3 months of pregnancy). However, there is no need to panic—most of this bothersome fluid will be lost during and shortly after your baby's delivery.

Try to make yourself more comfortable for the effects of edema:

➤ Lay down with your feet elevated on a pillow.

➤ Remove all of your tight rings.

➤ Wear loose comfortable shoes.

➤ Ease up on the salty stuff like sauerkraut, pickles, soy sauce, salty pretzels, and chips.

➤ *Never* restrict your fluid intake—always continue to drink plenty of fluids.

Oh My Aching Heart

Contrary to the name, *heartburn* is actually a burning sensation in your lower esophagus that is usually accompanied by a sour taste. Although this *lovely* feeling can happen at any time during your pregnancy, it's most common toward the last few months, when your baby is rapidly growing and exerting pressure on your stomach and uterus. What's more, during pregnancy, the valve between your stomach and esophagus can become relaxed making it easy for the food to occasionally reverse directions.

Some simple remedies to ease heartburn:

➤ Relax and eat your food slowly.

➤ Instead of eating a lot at one sitting, eat several smaller meals throughout the day.

➤ Limit fluids *with* meals, but increase fluids *between* meals.

➤ Chew gum or suck candy. Of course your dentist will hate me, but it can help to neutralize the acid.

➤ Never lie flat after you have eaten. In fact, keep your head elevated when you sleep with the help of extra pillows, and by placing a couple of books underneath the mattress to help tilt it slightly upward.

➤ Avoid wearing tight clothing. Stick with items that are loose and comfortable.

➤ Stand up and walk around. This can help encourage your gastric juices to flow in the right direction.

➤ Keep a log and track some foods that may be triggering your heartburn. Some common culprits include; coffee, colas, spicy foods, greasy fried foods, chocolate, citrus fruits and juices, and tomato-based products.

➤ *Never* take any antacids without your doctor's approval.

The Least You Need to Know

➤ You'll need an extra 55,000–80,000 calories during the entire 9-month haul! That's about 150 extra cals each day during the first trimester, and around 350 extra cals each day during the second and third trimesters.

➤ Extra protein, calcium, iron, and a variety of other nutrients are required through-out your pregnancy to cover the increased demands of the growing fetus.

➤ Healthy, normal weight women should aim for a 25–35 pound weight gain.

➤ Although nausea, constipation, water retention, and heartburn can be quite un-pleasant, rest assured they are generally normal side effects of pregnancy.

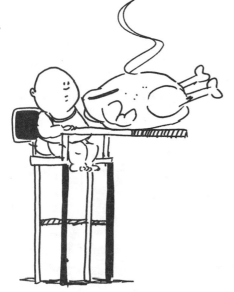

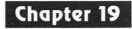

Move and Groove with a Bun in the Oven

Way back in the olden days (you know, when our parents had us) pregnancy was a time for rest—not exercise. (Say, you're pregnant? Relax, put your feet up, and have a few bon bons.) Today we know better. In fact, research reports that pregnant women who regularly exercise tend to have less aches and pains, better self esteem, more stamina, strength, and energy, and *perhaps* less fear of the delivery room.

Okay, so pregnancy is *not* the time to try to beat the world record in the high jump, or make your best time in the New York City marathon, but you can certainly continue with a modified version of your regular exercise regimen, or, if you're a newcomer to the world of fitness, begin a prenatal exercise program. Go ahead and compare delivering a baby to participating in an Olympic event. The nine-month pregnancy process is your chance to train for the big day. And hey, since "we moms" constantly compete *and* win at this intense event, I'm thinking that each and every one of us should get a gold medal placed around our necks as soon as the baby pops out.

Most Doctors Give the Green Light for Exercise

Most obstetricians today are keen on the idea of pregnant women exercising their way to the delivery room within the limits of common sense, of course. However, because certain medical instances rule out exercise, and nobody knows you medically better than your obstetrician, *never* begin exercising without first discussing it with your personal physician.

Q and A

Can you first begin an exercise program when you're pregnant—even if you're totally out of shape?

Yes! In fact, studies report that beginners can safely reap the benefits from exercise so long as they take it easy, appropriately warm up and cool down, keep their heart rates within a safe range, and have appropriate supervision for at *least* the first few sessions. Furthermore, fitness novices particularly must *always* get the okay from their docs before jumping in.

Q and A

Do fit women have easier deliveries than unfit women?

I hate to say it, but probably no. The bottom line is that an easy delivery most likely has to do with genetics, the positioning of the baby, and lots of luck! I've heard about "super fit" women with labors from hell, and I've heard about sedentary women popping out babies with just four pushes. Go figure. However, one thing is for sure, *fit* moms can better handle prolonged, agonizing labor, *and* bounce back with a quicker recoup period than unfit moms.

Let's Take a Look at What the Experts Say

This is a summary of the appropriate guidelines and recommendations from the American College of Obstetricians and Gynecologists (ACOG) on exercise during pregnancy and postpartum.

For healthy pregnant women, who do *not* have any additional risk factors, ACOG recommends the following:

1. During pregnancy, women can continue to exercise and derive health benefits even from mild to moderate exercise routines. Regular exercise—at least three times per week—is preferable to intermittent activity.

2. Avoid exercise in the supine position (lying on your back) after the first trimester. This position can decrease the cardiac output (blood flow) to the uterus. Also, avoid prolonged periods of motionless standing.

3. Pregnant women have less oxygen available for aerobic activity, and therefore should *not* expect to be able to do what they did pre-pregnancy. Pay close attention to your body's cues, and modify your exercise intensity according to how you feel. Always stop exercising when you feel fatigued and *never* push your body to exhaustion!

   Although some women may be able to continue with their regular weight-bearing exercises at the same intensity as they did pre-pregnancy, non-weight-bearing exercises such as swimming and biking may be easier to do and present less risk of injury.

4. Your changing size, shape, and weight can make certain exercises difficult, therefore avoid activities that can throw off your balance and possibly cause you to fall. Further, any type of exercise involving the potential for even mild abdominal trauma should be avoided.

5. Pregnancy requires an additional 300 calories a day. Thus, women who exercise during pregnancy should be particularly careful to ensure an adequate diet.

6. Pregnant women who exercise in the first trimester should stay cool by drinking plenty of water, wear appropriate clothing, and avoid very humid or hot environments.

7. Resume your pre-pregnancy exercise routines *gradually* after giving birth. Many of the physical changes that take place during pregnancy persist for four to six weeks.

You should *NOT* exercise during pregnancy if you have any of the following conditions:

➤ Pregnancy-induced hypertension (high blood pressure)

➤ Preterm rupture of membranes

➤ Preterm labor during the prior and/or current pregnancy

➤ Incompetent cervix/cerclage (a surgical procedure to close the cervix to keep the fetus intact in utero)

➤ Persistent second or third trimester bleeding

➤ Intrauterine growth retardation

In addition, women with certain other medical or obstetric conditions, including chronic hypertension or active thyroid, cardiac, vascular, or pulmonary disease, should be evaluated carefully in order to determine whether an exercise program is appropriate.

Warming Up, Cooling Down, and All the Stuff in the Middle

Pregnant or not, the ABC's of exercise remain the same. Be sure to begin each session with an appropriate *warm up*—some light aerobic activity that will rev up your system and prepare your body for the exercise to follow. Next, continue with a low-moderate intensity aerobic segment and be sure to pay close attention to your body's cues. During pregnancy, work at a comfortable pace, stop when you feel fatigued, and *never* push yourself to exhaustion. Lastly, always end your aerobic session with a proper *cooldown*— gradually slow down the pace to bring your heart rate back down to a resting level. See Chapter 13 for further details on exercise programs.

Stretch Your Bod—Carefully

Regular consistent stretching can help to maintain your flexibility, *and* prevent some of the usual pregnancy muscle tightness that typically sneaks up on you during the last trimester. Like always, stretching must proceed some type of warm up activity to increase your circulation and internal body temperature. Also, be sure to ease into each stretch gradually and hold for 10–30 seconds—*never* bounce! During pregnancy, the object is to stretch nice and easy. Don't ever push a stretch past the point of your pain-free range of motion.

Keep a Check on the Intensity

As of 1994, the American College of Obstetricians and Gynecologists (ACOG) lifted the rule that limited pregnant exercisers to working at a heart rate of 140 beats per minute, or less. Today, there are no limitations on heart rate. In fact, the experts say that you can monitor your own intensity as long as you exercise common sense. Keep in mind, you should *always* be able to comfortably carry on a conversation to ensure you are working in a safe aerobic range, and *never* push through fatigue, cramping, or any other discomfort. (Review the section on checking your heart rate in Chapter 13.)

Understand that being pregnant means you will typically fatigue more easily. Therefore, pre-plan to be cautious in the gym and modify your pre-pregnancy routine by decreasing both workout intensity *and* length. Also, don't expect to keep up with those nonpregnant jocks—go ahead and find yourself some less competitive opponents!

Q and A

What Should I Expect During The 1st, 2nd, and 3rd Trimesters?

During the first trimester, although size is not the issue, your raging hormones are! Because some women feel incredibly tired and queasy, listen to your body and do whatever activity you can manage until you feel better.

During the second trimester most women bounce back and feel like themselves again. If you feel up to it, this is a terrific time to incorporate regular exercise into your weekly schedule.

During the last trimester your growing waistline and weight may affect your stamina, agility, and balance, and you should think about switching to gentler activities that won't place strain on your joints and body (for instance, swimming and walking).

"Energize" Without All the Slamming and Jamming!

When it comes to selecting the *type* of exercise, every woman is different. Where one woman may be perfectly okay with modifying her usual sport (for instance, a runner may continue to jog at a slower pace), other women are not comfortable with all the jarring and jolting impact on the joints—especially in the last trimester, when your weight begins to climb. Think about switching to activities that are gentler to your system; for instance, walk instead of run, swim instead of high impact aerobics, or start pedaling on a stationary bike.

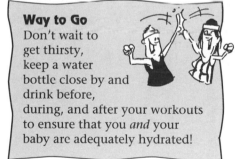

Way to Go
Don't wait to get thirsty, keep a water bottle close by and drink before, during, and after your workouts to ensure that you *and* your baby are adequately hydrated!

Take a Walk with Your "Babe"

Some of the great things about walking include the fact that there's no crashing impact, you can select your own pace and distance, you get quality "think time" (soon to be a commodity after the baby arrives), and walking can be done just about anywhere. For some fresh air, go for a trek around the neighborhood or hit a scenic trail. If you prefer the indoors, try a treadmill, or wander about your local shopping mall. Anything goes, just remember these key points:

➤ You need to keep a strong upright posture—lead with your chest.

➤ Rhythmically move your arms forward and back from the shoulders. Do not swing them higher than your chest or across your midline.

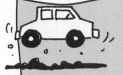

Rocky Road
Reduce your risk for injury by avoiding activities that require lots of balance and coordination because as your body shifts, so does your center of gravity due to your enlarged belly, breasts, and uterus.

Back off from things that may land you on the floor: skiing, horseback riding, biking, and skating.

Avoid sports that involve sharp, jerky movements like swinging a tennis racket, volleyball, bowling, and so on.

Resources
Try wearing two sports bras for some additional support and comfort of enlarged breasts.

Resources
Pick up some of these prenatal exercise tapes at your local video store and workout in the privacy of your own home.

➤ *Buns of Steel 8, Pregnancy Workout*

➤ *Denise Austine's Pregnancy Plus Workout*

➤ *Kathy Smith's Pregnancy Workout*

➤ Do not walk outdoors when the ground is icy. Remember, your balance is not as keen as it used to be.

➤ Don't try to conquer steep hills that can send your heart rate soaring, or place a lot of stress on your back.

➤ Do not walk in steamy, hot, or humid weather.

➤ Keep your body and baby well hydrated. Drink before, during, and after your walk.

➤ Eat a snack before you start off on your walk to prevent a drop in your blood sugar.

➤ Wear comfortable shoes with good support. Some women's feet swell during pregnancy, so you may need to wear shoes or sneaks at least a half size bigger.

➤ Wear appropriate clothing depending on the weather. On cold days wear layers that can be shed and tied around your waist as you begin to heat up.

Sign Up for a Prenatal Exercise Class

Prenatal exercise classes are specially designed for expectant moms, and take into consideration your shifting center of gravity, reduced stamina, and ever-changing bod! Generally, these specialty classes focus on thorough warm ups, cool downs, aerobic workouts, and stretching. In some instances, they may also include strength training and yoga. All exercises are carefully adapted and choreographed to keep you energized, but in a comfortable and appropriate fashion. Furthermore, you won't feel self-conscious since everyone in the class is in the same boat—give or take a few inches (or yards) around the waste. In other words, it's highly unlikely that the woman standing next to you will be wearing a thong leotard (*and if she is—more power to her*). It's also a nice place to bond, swap pregnancy war stories, and meet other women who are soon to have kids the same age as your own.

You can typically find out what's available in your area by checking with the local health clubs, hospitals, birthing centers, *or* you may even ask at your obstetrician's office.

Q and A

What the heck are Kegals?

These are exercises to strengthen the muscles within the pelvic floor (sort of deep inside, between your vagina and belly button). To figure out where these muscles are, try to stop and start your urine flow when your sitting on the toilet. Once you have located them, regularly strengthen your pelvic floor muscles with tightening and relaxing exercises. Pull upward and inward towards the body's midline, hold for about 5–10 seconds, and then relax. Repeat for as many times as you can, as often as you are willing. Kegal exercises can be done sitting, standing, or lying down, and can drastically help to increase genital circulation, strengthen and maintain the pelvic floor muscles, and prevent incontinence after the baby is born.

Yes, "Moms-to-Be" Can Lift Weights

Being pregnant doesn't necessarily mean passing up the weight room. In fact, incorporating some light weight training into your pregnancy schedule may possibly cut back on some of the back and shoulder pain associated with enlarged breasts, extra weight, and a growing uterus. What's more, it may also reduce the leg cramps and neck strain that some women experience toward the last trimester. Personally, my favorite benefit from prenatal lifting is that your muscles will be primed for the "baby *aftermath.*" That is, ready to lug around your pocketbook, diaper bag, and stroller on one arm, while carrying your baby on the other. To this day, I still amaze my sister Debra with the amount of equipment I can juggle with just two arms!

If you are experienced with weights, you can go ahead and continue with a *modified* version of your regular routine (adjust the amount of weight and number of reps to how you feel). However, if you are a novice with the dumbbells and machines this is definitely *not* the time to lift anything unsupervised. You can ask a qualified trainer who is experienced with pregnant women to show you the ropes.

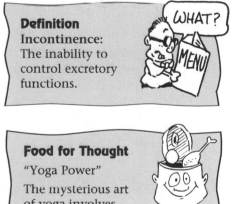

Definition
Incontinence: The inability to control excretory functions.

Food for Thought
"Yoga Power"
The mysterious art of yoga involves breathing, relaxation, stretching, and body awareness. Therefore, yoga can play a magical role in making you feel terrific *during* and *after* your pregnancy.

Some Things to Consider:

➤ Regroup your weight training goals. Instead of focusing on intense workouts that will increase strength and define your muscles, relax, take it easy, and simply concentrate on strength maintenance.

➤ Because you may become less agile and coordinated due to the extra weight you are carrying, consider sticking with the machines. They offer much more support and require less balance than the free weights.

➤ Be aware that some machines require inappropriate positioning, and as your belly expands in front, you *literally* may not be able to fit on some of the machines comfortably (Ah, isn't pregnancy fun?). But don't let that halt the workout, ask a trainer to show you some safe (perhaps non-machine) exercises. Or simply forget about that particular exercise until you are back into your post-pregnancy routine again.

➤ The amount of weight you should lift depends *both* on your strength pre-pregnancy, *and* how you are feeling *during* your pregnancy. Lift what feels slightly challenging during the last few reps but *not* an amount that really pushes your limit.

➤ Pay close attention to your form and concentrate on smooth and steady breathing.

➤ Don't be discouraged if you have to cut back on the weights as you get further into your pregnancy. In fact, expect to cut back. Remember, you're pregnant—not Wonder Woman. Women typically get more tired, and have less agility and balance toward the end of the 9-month term.

➤ If at any point you feel nauseous, dizzy, overly fatigued, or any other uncomfortable sensation (cramping, knotting, tingling, etc.), stop exercising IMMEDIATELY and speak with your doctor before continuing.

Q and A

Can I lie on my back and do sit-ups?

Yes, but only during the first trimester. After the fourth month you risk pinching off the inferior vena cava, an important large vein that carries blood back to the heart. During pregnancy, the weight of your growing uterus may compress this vein and cause you to feel faint. Instead of stomach exercises on your back, ask a trainer to show you how to work your abdominals on your side or standing up.

Bouncing Back After the Baby Arrives

Generally, five to six weeks *after* delivering your bundle of joy, your doctor will give you the okay to resume all exercise. A task that is easier said than done. Between the sleep deprivation and feeling like your body's been through a war, merely scheduling in the time and getting up the motivation is a feat in itself. But take a deep breath and try to round up some energy because exercise can do wonders for both your mind and body. Just start off slow, go at your own pace, and *gradually* ease back into your pre-pregnancy routine.

> **Resources**
> Pick up *Fit Pregnancy* magazine and get all the latest scoop on keeping fit while you're expecting. It's from the folks over at *Shape* magazine and hits the news-stands three to four times each year.

The Least You Need to Know

➤ Women who regularly exercise during pregnancy tend to have less aches and pains, better self esteem, and more stamina, strength, and energy.

➤ Because some medical instances rule out exercise, *always* get the okay from your doctor before beginning an exercise program.

➤ Since pregnancy generally reduces your stamina, speed, and agility, expect to modify your pre-pregnancy routines by decreasing your workout *intensity* and *length*. Also, always keep your heart rate within a comfortable working range and *never* push your body to exhaustion.

➤ Most pregnant women prefer gentler activities that do not strain the joints such as swimming, walking, and stationary bikes—especially during the last trimester when your girth and weight start to climb.

➤ Drink plenty of water before, during, and after exercise to ensure that you and your baby are well-hydrated.

Part 6
Healthy Kids: From the Cradle to College Graduation

As a mother and nutritionist, I understand that sometimes it can become quite a challenge to get your kids to eat healthy. If we could only mold carrots and bananas into log shapes and pop a "Snickers" wrapper on top, life would be so much simpler. Unfortunately for many parents, it's a lot tougher than that!

The first chapter in this section is dedicated to the younger folks. It offers creative suggestions for sneaking veggies into meals, making lower-fat after school snack ideas, and tips to encourage more physical activity. The second chapter addresses the college crowd and maps out the best bites in the campus dining hall, along with the real-deal on vending machines, late night munchies, alcohol and partying, and of course, how to avoid those notorious "freshman fifteen" pounds of weight that seem to creep up on a lot of college students.

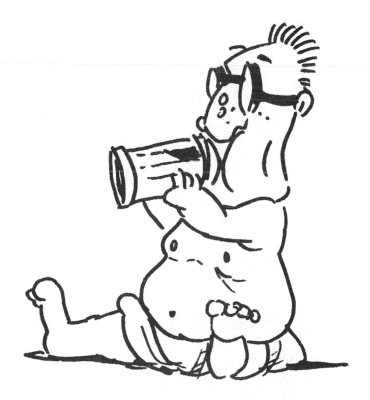

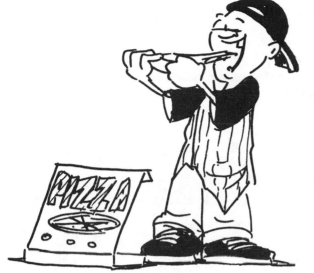

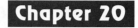

Chapter 20

From Pampers to Prom Night— Food for the Younger Folks

In This Chapter

➤ Foods for the first year of life

➤ Nutrition guidelines for growing kids

➤ Involving your kids in the kitchen

➤ Healthy snack-attacks

➤ Getting your couch potato to exercise

Being a kid these days is a pretty demanding job. Between homework, after-school activities, sports-teams, being popular, and keeping up with the latest fashion trends, it's *especially* important that the younger folks learn to keep their bodies fit and healthy so that they're better-equipped to take on the world.

As a mother, as well as a nutritionist, I understand that nobody knows your children better than you, the parent. Therefore, this chapter is *not* about telling you what you should and shouldn't feed your kids, but merely suggestions and guidelines to help assist you with your tremendous endeavor. Read on and learn how to encourage your kids to eat nutritious foods *and* get plenty of physical activity. Remember, healthy kids grow up to be healthy adults.

Your Very First Food Decision—Breast Milk or Formula?

Most pediatricians and nutritionists across the board agree that breast milk is the food of choice for growing babies. First off, nursing is a beautiful mother-baby bonding experience *and* it's economically savvy. In other words, it's cheap, cheap, cheap! But most importantly, breast milk has the capability to protect your baby from several infections since it is believed to carry immunities (protective substances) from mother to infant. In addition, *colostrum,* the yellowish pre-milk substance that is secreted in the first few days after delivery, may carry even *more* antibodies, plus it's loaded with protein and zinc.

> **Food for Thought**
> Have your child compare his or her body to a sports car. Fuel the car with high-quality gasoline and it will run smoothly. Fuel the car with watered-down gas and it poops out. Your body works the same way: fuel your system with smart food choices from all of the foods on the food guide pyramid, and you'll feel terrific. On the other hand, eat lots of junk food and, like the car, you'll poop out.

But for all you women who choose not to nurse, or aren't able to nurse, don't lose any sleep. Companies today make sophisticated baby formulas that closely mimic the components in human milk. What's more, babies that are formula-fed can receive just as much "snuggling time" as babies that are breast-fed, and therefore form close bonds with mom. So whichever you decide (the bottle or the breast), rest assured *all* kids can have a shot at getting into Harvard University, and/or making the Olympic soccer team!

When and How to Start Solids

Although, you may choose to nurse way past six months, at this point your growing baby will need more calories and iron than breast milk or formulas alone can supply. Generally, pediatricians recommend beginning with solid foods between four and six months. Here's some strategies for getting started.

> ➤ A general rule of thumb is to introduce only one new food at a time (over the course of four to six days) to rule out food allergies and intolerances. If your baby tolerates a food, and you don't notice any adverse reactions (i.e., skin rashes, wheezing, diarrhea, stomach aches), you can graduate on to the next food item. Highly allergic foods include wheat, egg white, and cow's milk. Avoid giving these to your child until seven-to-nine months old.

> ➤ Rice cereal is usually recommended for the first food introduction since it is the least allergenic. Follow the directions on the cereal box (usually 3-5 Tablespoons of dry cereal is mixed with breast milk, formula or water) Although, it may seem bland to you, *don't* add anything else—no sugar, salt, honey, etc. Your baby will find it perfectly fine, and it's really the texture that you want him or her to get used to.

➤ After cereal has passed the test, try some plain yogurt, pureed fruit, and pureed veggies. Watch how your baby starts to master the art of pushing the food back into the mouth with the tongue—what a genius! You can also give your baby unsweetened 100% fruit juice at this point, but be sure to dilute it to half-strength with water.

➤ By six to ten months your baby's digestive system is maturing and it's time to introduce all sorts of mashed concoctions. Try strained meats, chicken, turkey, cottage cheese, egg yolks (avoid egg whites since they tend to be highly allergenic), and mashed lentils and beans.

➤ By 12 months you can go ahead and substitute regular cow's milk for formula, with the okay from your pediatrician. Encourage at least three full cups of milk per day, but not so much more that your child will be too full for any solid foods that supply the necessary calories and iron.

➤ Remember to go at your own pace, and listen to what your pediatrician has to say about the growth and development of your little one— clearly the best indication of your baby's nutritional status.

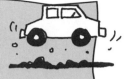

Rocky Road
Don't be over-zealous about buying "low-fat" foods for your infant. Although a good practice for older children, the first two years of life require *extra* calories and fat for proper growth and development! So stick with the whole-fat dairy until your child turns two years old, *or* your pediatrician says otherwise.

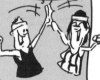

Way to Go
Tips for feeding your little one.

Make mealtime relaxed and pleasur-able. Don't try to rush through your baby's meals in five minutes flat, *or* juggle the phone in one hand and spoon in the other. Go at your baby's pace, and allow him or her to touch the food and try to bring it up to the mouth. Constantly engage in conversation, smiles, and positive feedback.

Popular First Year Foods

rice cereals	barley cereals	oat cereals
squash	sweet potato	carrots
green beans	peas	avocado
yogurt, plain	applesauce	bananas
peaches	plums	pears
chicken	beef	lamb
turkey		

Rocky Road

Watch out for certain foods. During the first year, avoid foods that are difficult to chew and can possibly cause choking like nuts, popcorn, hard candy, and raw carrots. Also avoid foods that have tough outer skins, such as grapes and hot dogs, and foods that are thick and sticky such as peanut butter.

Honey should definitely be avoided in children under one year of age since it can cause infant botulism. Honey is sometimes contaminated with spores of clostridium botulinum and in an infant's intestine, these spores can grow and produce a toxin which can make a baby sick and—in extreme cases—cause death. Adults need not worry because "friendly" bacteria present in their intestines prevents these spores from growing.

Be extra cautious when introducing foods which tend to be highly allergenic such as egg whites, wheat, corn, nuts, seafood, citrus fruits, chocolate, cocoa, seafood, pork, berries, and tomatoes. In some instances your pediatrician may tell you to hold off until after the first year.

The Right Stuff for Growing Kids

These are the basic guidelines for children three-years and older. Keep in mind, that this chart represents the *minimum* requirements—*all* kids require at least this amount. Obviously, active kids who participate in after-school sports (or kids that just plain run around a lot) will need much more food than the average couch potato. Also, expect the portions sizes to vary. Younger children generally eat much smaller portions than older kids.

Food Group	Minimum Servings/Day	Key Nutrients
Bread and grain group	6+	Carbohydrates, B-vitamins, iron
Vegetable group	3+	vitamin C, vitamin A, folic acid, magnesium, fiber
Fruit group	2+	vitamin C, vitamin A, potassium, fiber
Milk, yogurt, and cheese group	3+	calcium, riboflavin, protein
Meat, poultry, dried beans, eggs, and nuts group	2	protein, B-vitamins iron, zinc

Q and A

Should I worry if my kids aren't getting enough food?

No. Children generally eat when they are hungry, and stop when they are full. You may, however, want to pay attention to daily food choices among various food groups. If certain foods are consistently left out, try to brainstorm on ways to work them into the day.

Be a Healthy Role Model

Monkey see, monkey do! As your children grow they observe and copy everything you do—*eating habits included*. Remember, actions speak much louder than words, so start munching on those fruits and vegetables. Teach your kids the food groups with fun meal creations.

Cook With Your Kids, Not for Them!

Introduce your kids to healthy eating *and* the kitchen! I've found that children are more interested and *willing* to eat unfamiliar foods when they have personally participated in the preparation. Try some of the following suggestions:

Way to Go
Make mealtime fun for your *younger* kids, set a place at the dinner table for a special doll or stuffed animal.

➤ Select a few nights each week and involve your kids with dinner planning *and* preparation. Designate different jobs for each child.

➤ You may prefer to single out one child at a time. For instance, Tuesday night may be the night you and your son whip up a creative dinner concoction for the family. Thursday night may be a special night for just you and your daughter to plan the evening spread.

Food for Thought
Up until the age of 24 years, kids are laying down the foundation for a lifetime of strong, healthy bones, so be sure to eat and drink plenty of low-fat dairy along with buying calcium-fortified juices and other food products that are out on the market today. For more info see Chapter 8.

➤ How about an entire "theme night?" For example, one night may be Japanese. Make chicken teriyaki over rice, you can set up a table on the floor, sit on pillows, and use chopsticks instead of forks. Or, make it Greek night and serve Greek salads while wearing togas.

Fun and Easy Recipes

Here are a few recipes that will help your kids enjoy cooking.

Breakfast Berry Crepes

Serves four

2 cups whole-grain flour

1 egg, beaten

2 $^1/_2$ cups low-fat milk

non-stick vegetable spray

$^1/_2$ cup blueberries

$^1/_2$ cup raspberries

$^1/_2$ sliced strawberries

Place flour in a bowl and add egg plus 2 cups of milk (save $^1/_2$ cup). Beat with a wire whisk until all lumps are gone and the mixture is completely smooth. Gradually add the remaining $^1/_2$ cup of milk to make a thin batter. Use non-stick cooking spray on hot skillet (medium-high temp), and pour enough batter in the pan just to make a large circle. Sprinkle desired amount of fruit on top and press down into the crepe. Cook for approx. 2–3 more minutes and then flip the crepe and cook the other side. Carefully lift onto a plate and roll it all the way up.

*From the kitchen of Lisa Alexander and Jesse Bauer

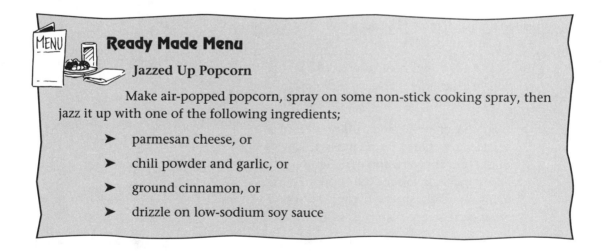

Ready Made Menu

Jazzed Up Popcorn

Make air-popped popcorn, spray on some non-stick cooking spray, then jazz it up with one of the following ingredients;

➤ parmesan cheese, or

➤ chili powder and garlic, or

➤ ground cinnamon, or

➤ drizzle on low-sodium soy sauce

Tuna Salad Cones

Serves four

Open a can of water-packed tuna and drain off liquid. Mash up tuna and mix in grated carrots, chopped tomatoes, and some shredded low-fat cheddar cheese (optional). Lightly mix with low-fat mayonnaise *or* Italian salad dressing, and scoop into flat-bottomed ice cream cones (not the sugar kind). Serve for lunch or at a party, your kids will love them!

*From the kitchen of Lisa, Jason, and Harley Bauer

"Have a Blast With Your Blender"

Banana-Berry Frosty

1 cup low-fat milk	2 teaspoons vanilla
1 cup of fresh strawberries	3–4 ice cubes
1 banana	

Place all ingredients into the blender and mix until smooth and fluffy.

Peanut Butter-Yogurt Milkshake

4 big scoops of vanilla frozen yogurt (or any flavor you prefer)	1–2 Tablespoons peanut butter
1 cup low-fat milk	

Mix all ingredients in the blender until thick and smooth.

No Such Thing as "Forbidden" Foods

Clearly there are healthier foods than others; however, there is room in every meal plan for *all* foods, even the junky stuff! Create a positive attitude about food by emphasizing healthy choices and limiting (*not eliminating*) the not-so-healthy cakes, cookies, and candy. In fact, forbidding your kids to eat certain foods doesn't work, it only makes the high-fat stuff that much more enticing.

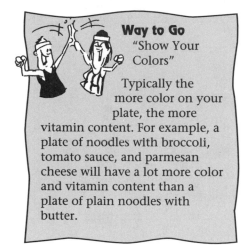

Way to Go
"Show Your Colors"

Typically the more color on your plate, the more vitamin content. For example, a plate of noodles with broccoli, tomato sauce, and parmesan cheese will have a lot more color and vitamin content than a plate of plain noodles with butter.

One approach is to introduce young children to the food guide pyramid and explain the importance of fueling your body with the various food groups, *then* limit the desserty foods to one per day. This can even work for overweight kids. Instead of taking away *all* desserts, simply focus on *increasing* fruits, vegetables, and physical activity. Remember, a weight problem is *not* from eating a slice of cake or a few cookies. It's usually from lack of exercise and *excessive* amounts of these fats and sweets.

And what about your teenagers? As your kids grow up, you tend to have much less control over what they eat. Continue to encourage healthy food choices and certainly downplay the unhealthy stuff—but be careful *not* to create an obsessive environment of "bad food/good food"—it can backfire into a serious eating disorder.

The Sneaky Gourmet: 15 Ways to Disguise Vegetables

Say your child won't go near vegetables? See if you can sneak in a few here and there with some of these suggestions.

1. Add a mixed vegetable medley into your meatloaf recipe.

2. Scatter cooked vegetables throughout pasta and then cover with marinara sauce.

3. Grate carrots into tuna fish salad or chicken salad and stuff in a pita pocket.

4. Make homemade pizza. Toss on sliced mushrooms and chopped broccoli *before* spreading on the cheese.

5. Make vegetable lasagna. You can stick with a single vegetable like spinach (*see* Spinach Lasagna recipe in Chapter 17), *or* mix in a variety of chopped, cooked vegetables such as zucchini, cauliflower, broccoli, carrots, mushrooms, green beans, and so on.

6. Add cooked peas, corn and carrots into mashed potatoes.

7. Serve vegetable soup with crackers.

8. Puree cooked squash and carrots, then add small amounts into your ground beef or ground turkey. Shape into hamburgers or turkey-burgers and cook on the grill.

9. Top a baked potato with chopped broccoli and low-fat melted cheese.

10. Make low-fat zucchini and carrot muffins.

11. Serve "make-your-own tacos" and have different stations set up with lean ground beef (or ground turkey), sliced tomatoes, shredded lettuce, and carrots.

12. Make chicken-vegetable kabobs. Alternate chunks of *grilled* chicken, peppers, tomatoes, onions, zucchini, and mushrooms on metal skewers. Set up a variety of dips that your kids can have fun experimenting with such as barbecue sauce, honey mustard sauce, sweet and sour sauce, and low-fat salad dressings. Of course, maybe you'll get lucky and your kids will simply like the original marinade.

13. Finely chop cooked broccoli and thoroughly mix into your rice.

14. Turn your kids on to wok cooking and have them assist with washing and cutting up the vegetables. Try chicken-vegetable stir-fry, beef-vegetable stir-fry, or seafood-vegetable stir-fry. Pour them all over rice or linguini and hand out the chopsticks.

15. Make a spinach dip with low-fat plain yogurt, low-fat sour cream, and pureed cooked spinach. Have them dip carrots, celery, peppers, and zucchini slices. If they don't want to dip with raw veggies give them some crackers—at least they'll get the spinach from the dip.

Resources
Unfortunately enough, recent studies report 21% of 12 to 19-year-old American kids are obese. That's a pretty alarming considering that obesity can seriously hinder socialization *plus* lead to a slew of serious medical problems including heart disease.

Turn Off that Tube!

Too much television generally means too much sitting around. Try and put a two-hour limit on TV watching and encourage your kids to get up and move! Teach them about the importance of exercise and have them do something physical everyday for at least 30 minutes. Have them walk the dog, jump rope, roller blade, throw a ball around, swim, play tag, play basketball, sign up for an after-school class, *or* join a sports team.

Healthy After-school Snack-Attacks:

Fresh fruit

Veggies and low-fat dip

Yogurt and granola

Fig bars and low-fat milk

Fruit cocktail in light syrup

Bananas and apple slices with peanut butter

Carrots and celery with peanut butter

Whole-wheat toast with apple butter

Trail mix (nuts and raisins)

Dried fruit

Cereal with fruit and low-fat milk

English muffin pizzas

Frozen fruit bars

Frozen yogurt pops

Banana-Berry frosty (see sidebox recipe)

Peanut butter-Yogurt milkshake (see sidebox recipe)

Animal crackers and graham crackers

Pretzels and fruit juice

Vegetable soup and pita

Flavored rice cakes

Jazzed up popcorn (see sidebox recipes)

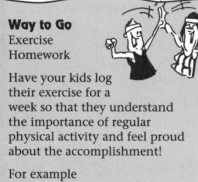

Way to Go
Exercise
Homework

Have your kids log their exercise for a week so that they understand the importance of regular physical activity and feel proud about the accomplishment!

For example
Monday: Rode my bike for 1 hour
Tuesday: dance class for 45 minutes

Resources
For further reading pick up *How to Teach Nutrition to Your Kids* By Connie Liakos Evers, MS RD Carrot Press 1-800-291-6098

The Least You Need to Know

➤ Most health experts recommend breast-milk over formula since breast-milk is believed to pass protective substances from mother to baby.

➤ Typically between four and six months, your pediatrician will give you the okay to start your baby on solids. Stick with one food at a time to rule out food allergies.

➤ All growing kids should eat a daily total of *at least* 6 servings of breads and grains, 2 servings of fruit, 3 servings of veggies, 3 servings of dairy, and 2 servings of meat, poultry, dried beans, fish, eggs, or nuts. Expect younger kids to eat *much* smaller serving sizes than older children.

➤ Let kids be kids, and occasionally eat junk food. Understand that an obsessive environment of denial can backfire.

➤ Put a two hour limit to television watching and encourage your kids to become more physically active.

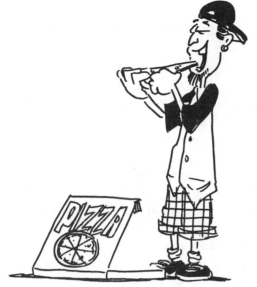

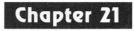
Eating Through the College Years

Does this routine sound familiar? The day begins with no breakfast—"who has time?" With an English class at 8A.M., you are lucky if you can get dressed, brush your teeth, and run out the door. Breakfast is just *not* a priority. By lunch time, you are delirious with hunger and ready to fall off your feet. Food card in hand (no money needed and all the food you can eat, *what a concept!*), you are off and running to the campus dining hall. Lunch consists of a cheeseburger, French-fries, and a cola, topped off with chocolate cake or a donut (gotta keep up that strength you know, two more grueling classes ahead). By 6 P.M., you stumble back into the dining hall, exhausted from your chaotic day. You find yourself loading your tray with anything that looks appealing: fried chicken and mashed potatoes, burritos and sour cream, or pepperoni pizza, of course washed down with another cola. And hey, since it's all free, why not grab a few cookies and a soft-serve ice cream cone before heading back to the dorm.

It is time to face the music—you need a nutrition tune-up!

Mistake 1: No Time for Breakfast

It's ironic to think that after all these years, mom was actually right. Eating breakfast *is* important. Unfortunately though, many college students make it a habit to skip this essential meal. Remember, when you wake up from a good night's sleep, your body has been in a fasting state for at least eight hours. Unless, of course, there was a late night party, then we may be talking about two hours sleep! As I've mentioned earlier in the book, "Break-Fast" in the morning helps kick your system into gear by supplying energy in the form of food to your body. Without any food, you would become tired, sluggish, and probably fight to stay awake during morning classes. Have you ever had to literally hold your eyelids open with your fingers while your teacher was lecturing at 8 A.M.? Fueling your body with a healthy breakfast can keep you alert and focused during your morning schedule.

Skipping Breakfast to "Save Calories?"...I Don't Think So!

By the way, for all you students who skip breakfast to "save calories," think again. The majority of breakfast skippers wind up so ravenous by lunch time and dinner that they overcompensate and pig-out. Here's an example of how not eating breakfast can become a diet disaster: Nancy, a student at University of Michigan, skipped breakfast regularly to try and lose weight. She would then find herself so famished by lunch time that she would inevitably over-eat—and of course sabotage her diet in the process. I recommended that she experiment with a healthy breakfast for two weeks to determine if eating in the morning would help control her midday munchies. Sure enough, she felt more energetic and alert during her morning routine, and ate *substantially* less at lunch, enabling her to lose three pounds. No time for breakfast? MAKE THE TIME.

Mistake 2: Too Many High-Fat Food Choices

For many people, going off to college is their first time away from home. It's not easy having to constantly fend for yourself when your used to the luxury of mom's home cooking. Oh, the memories of a stocked fridge, fresh fruit, and hot meals placed out on the dinner table each night.

Hey, just because you're on your own, there's no reason to slouch off in the food department. Most of the foods mentioned above in the "college scenario from hell," are loaded with fat, sugar, and salt, which can lead to a host of problems, including weight gain and other serious illnesses. Furthermore, these foods lack vitamins, minerals, and other essential nutrients that your body needs to function properly.

You say it's impossible to eat right at school? That your college food service doesn't provide any healthy foods? Sure it does, you just need to look beyond some of the junky stuff. There's actually a great deal of good in your school dining hall. Where else can you have everything from soup to nuts at your fingertips, three meals a day? Read on and learn to choose foods that will make you look and feel your best all the time.

Making the Grade in the Campus Dining Hall

The following is a collection of food stations commonly found in university dining halls. Find the stations that your school offers, and learn to ace the test, with nutritious choices at breakfast, lunch, and dinner.

CEREAL BARS: There is nothing quicker and more satisfying than a bowl of cereal in the morning. Enjoy both the hot and cold varieties, they are high in carbohydrates, chock-full of nutrients, and generally very low in fat.

CHOOSE MORE OFTEN   First, choose high-fiber cereals such as All-Bran, Raisin Bran, Bran Flakes, Bran Chex, or any others with the word "bran" in the name. Fiber not only relieves constipation, but also protects against certain cancers. Pour on plenty of low-fat milk or yogurt to boost your daily calcium, and don't forget to toss in lots of fresh fruit (bananas, peaches, blueberries, strawberries, apples, raisins, raspberries, pineapple, etc.) for extra vitamin content and added sweetness. Don't just stop at the cold cereals, warm up those cold winter mornings with a hearty bowl of hot oatmeal or cream of wheat.

CHOOSE LESS OFTEN   Forget about those sugary cereals. Although they are delicious, some brands actually pack more sugar into one serving than a piece of cake. If high sugar cereal is a must, try mixing it with a healthier cereal to reduce the amount of sugar. For example, mix half a bowl of Frosted Flakes with half a bowl of Bran flakes. Who knows, after a while, you may even prefer the healthier cereal. Avoid pouring on "whole fat" milk. It is loaded with artery clogging saturated fat. Try switching first to 2% milk, then 1%. Hey, if you're extra determined, go for the skim (no fat at all).

SALAD BARS: The word "salad" usually brings to mind an array of bright colored vegetables such as lettuce, tomatoes, cucumbers, carrots, onions, broccoli, peppers, etc. All of these salad ingredients offer vitamins, minerals, fiber, and—the best news of all— very few calories. Unfortunately, salad bars also offer a variety of high-fat side items which can turn your health conscious plate into a catastrophe! Read on, and "PASS" your next trip to the salad bar with flying colors.

CHOOSE MORE OFTEN   Pile your plate with lots of colorful raw vegetables. Jazz up your salad with protein and turn it into a meal. Throw on some chick peas, beans, eggs, low-fat cheeses, sliced turkey/roast beef, or plain tuna. Stick with a "light" or low-fat dressing, or use plenty of balsamic vinegar with a touch of oil. If regular dressing is a must, opt for vinaigrettes, or go easy on the higher fat selections (1–2 Tablespoons).

CHOOSE LESS OFTEN   Don't pile your plate with mayonnaise-laden side dishes such as macaroni salad, cole slaw, potato salad, and carrot-raisin salad. If your waistline cannot afford extra fat calories, beware of other high-fat side items such as oily pasta salads, cheese, olives, avocado, bacon bits, sunflower seeds, nuts, croutons, and creamy salad dressings.

HOT STATIONS: Ready to load your tray with whatever looks most delicious? Decisions, decisions, decisions! First, stop and figure out which entree and side dish will fit into your fat budget. Make savvy choices by understanding the healthier methods of meal preparation. Naturally, an occasional trek on the dark-side is O.K., but generally try to stick with the foods on the "CHOOSE MORE OFTEN" list.

CHOOSE MORE OFTEN   Look for entrees and side items that are grilled, baked, steamed, broiled, blackened, lightly stir-fried, mesquite-grilled, poached, and lightly marinated. Choose dishes made with teriyaki, soy sauce, barbecue sauce, tomato sauce, marinara sauce, honey-mustard sauce, white wine sauce, or broth. Although some of these sauces may be high in sugar and salt, they are far better choices than the "CHOOSE LESS OFTEN" list.

➤ Eat plenty of skinless chicken and turkey, and all types of seafood. Even an occasional portion of lean, red meat (2–3 times per week) can fit into a healthy eating plan. When selecting a soup, opt for non-creamy versions such as vegetable-barley, chicken-noodle, lentil-bean combos, tomato-rice, minestrone, manhattan clam chowder (the red, not the white), and garden-vegetable. Stick with nonfried side dishes, such as steamed or sautéed vegetables; corn-on-the-cob; mashed, baked, or roasted potatoes; rice; couscous; and pastas in light oil or red sauce.

➤ Be imaginative, and mix together several items that are offered to create your own original meal. For example, scoop rice into vegetable soups, mix vegetables into pastas, spread yogurt on a baked potato. The sky's the limit.

CHOOSE LESS OFTEN   Don't chow down on all of those fried favorites: fried chicken, fried fish, fried eggs, pan-fried burgers, French fries, onion rings, fried potato skins, hash browns, vegetable tempura, etc. Also stay away from entrees that are loaded with whole-milk cheese such as lasagna, baked ziti, cheesy burritos, chicken/veal/eggplant parmesan, grilled cheese sandwiches, macaroni and cheese, calzones, and cheesy pizza (especially with pepperoni, sausage, or meatball). Oh yeah, let's not forget those rich pasta sauces like Fettucini Alfredo (heart attack city!).

➤ Avoid creamy soups such as cream of broccoli, cream of mushroom, French onion soup (with cheese), New England clam chowder, and lobster bisque. Also beware of chicken skins and higher fat meats such as hot dogs, bacon, sausage, pepperoni, chicken wings, buffalo wings, and ribs. Limit the amount of eggs you eat for breakfast to twice per week. Although the whites are pure protein, the yolks contain too much cholesterol.

REFRIGERATOR ITEMS: Whoever said that a meal had to be hot anyway? There are lots of healthy options hidden in the refrigerator section of your dining hall. From sandwiches to prepared salads and yogurts, as long as you make smart choices, a "cold" meal can be nutritious and satisfying.

CHOOSE MORE OFTEN   Stick with lower-fat sandwiches such as turkey breast, grilled chicken, lean roast beef, and ham. Add some extra fiber by throwing on some veggies and choosing whole wheat bread over white bread. Stick with mustard, ketchup, or light salad dressing as a spread. Get into low-fat yogurts, they are loaded with calcium, protein, and generally tend to be low in calories. Prepared salads with chicken, turkey, roast beef, ham, and moderate amounts of cheese are also smart alternatives—just go easy on the dressing.

CHOOSE LESS OFTEN   Don't make it a habit to gobble down sandwiches loaded with globs of mayonnaise such as tuna salad, chicken salad, egg salad and seafood salad. Avoid pre-prepared sandwiches that contain high-fat meats such as salami, bologna, pepperoni, and bacon. Furthermore, limit the salads and sandwiches that come with a lot of extra cheese and oil.

BEVERAGES: Feel like a tall, cold glass of cola? *NOT!* With every beverage dispenser at your fingertips, why not select something healthier? The following guidelines provide you with best bets for quenching your thirst.

CHOOSE MORE OFTEN   Drink water, water, and more water! Plain old water may sound boring but it happens to be the "super hero" of all beverages. Not only is water the best way to quench your thirst and hydrate your body, it also helps to move things along (I think you get the picture). Try mixing club soda, seltzer, mineral water, or sparkling water with fresh lemon, lime, orange, or even some fruit juice for flavor.

➤ If H_2O doesn't thrill you, at least select a drink that offers you some nutrition rather than pure sugar. For example, natural fruit juices contain several vitamins such as A, C, potassium, magnesium, and other B-vitamins, depending on the type of juice. Low-fat milk and chocolate milk are also smart alternatives since they both provide calcium and protein.

CHOOSE LESS OFTEN   Don't guzzle down all of those sugary drinks (soda, fruit punch, and sugary iced teas) These are PURE SUGAR, NO NUTRITION. Diet beverages are not

249

such a bargain either, with all those artificial sweeteners, who needs them? Go easy on coffees and teas as well. With all that caffeine, you'll be jittery, irritable, and bouncing off the walls.

POTATO BARS: Take advantage of this no-fat complex carbohydrate and *MANGIA*. Not only are baked potatoes low in calories (about 100 cals for a medium potato), but they are loaded with potassium, and a decent amount of fiber if you eat the skin. Don't even think about glopping on the butter and sour cream (fat, fat, fat). Instead, try some of these healthier alternatives:

CHOOSE MORE OFTEN   Try a baked potato topped with:

Broccoli and marinara sauce

Vegetarian chili

Salsa, ketchup, or barbecue sauce

Low-fat yogurt (plain and flavored)

Stir-fried vegetables with soy sauce

Cottage cheese

Tossed salad and light vinaigrette

Dijon mustard

Cooked veggies and parmesan cheese

One pat of butter or margarine

> **Way to Go**
> The campus dining hall is loaded with *both* healthy and not so healthy foods.
> Bottom Line: Balance out your meals and select a variety of nutritious foods *most* of the time, and you can certainly sneak in some of the *"not so healthy stuff"* every once in a while. The key is to keep fat intake down (approx 30% of calories should come from fat) while eating a variety of foods from all of the food groups.

CHOOSE LESS OFTEN   You already know what I'm gonna say about this one. LAY OFF THE MOUNDS OF BUTTER AND SOUR CREAM

DESSERTS: The perfect ending to a meal—or maybe not!

CHOOSE MORE OFTEN   Select fresh fruit, frozen yogurt, Jell-O, angel-food cake, low-fat cookies, sorbet, frozen fruit bars, applesauce and baked apples. If you feel like going all out, *share* a decadent dessert with a friend.

CHOOSE LESS OFTEN   Don't make it a habit to top off each meal with a high-fat gloppy dessert such as chocolate cake, cookies, ice cream sundaes, strawberry shortcake, puddings, custards, and apple pie a la mode.

BREAKFAST IDEAS IN THE CAMPUS DINING HALL

CHOOSE MORE OFTEN

Low-fat milk, toast with jam, and an orange

Bowl of cereal, low-fat milk, banana, and orange juice

Yogurt with cereal and raisins, and a glass of milk or juice

Bagel with thin layer of cream cheese and tomato slices, glass of milk, and an apple

Oatmeal with sliced peaches and a glass of grapefruit juice

Pancakes with strawberries, bananas, and go "light" on the syrup with a glass of milk or hot tea with lemon

Waffle topped with peaches and yogurt and a glass of grapefruit juice

Scrambled eggs, bagel with jam, and a glass of orange juice

Vegetable omelet, fresh fruit salad, and a glass of milk

Poached eggs on a English muffin, light hot cocoa, and sliced melon

LUNCH IDEAS IN THE CAMPUS DINING HALL

CHOOSE MORE OFTEN

Turkey breast sandwich on whole wheat bread, carrot sticks, and frozen yogurt with granola

Bowl of lentil soup, a baked potato topped with broccoli and marinara sauce, and an orange

Vegetable pizza and fresh fruit salad

Hamburger on a bun, side salad, and an apple

Grilled chicken sandwich with lettuce, tomato, two cookies, and low-fat milk

Grilled vegetables with cheese in a pita pocket and fruit salad

Chicken noodle soup, low-fat yogurt, and a frozen fruit bar

Large tossed salad with beans and chickpeas, pita bread, and a low-fat fruit yogurt topped off with a pear

Salad with turkey breast, roll, and angel food cake topped with strawberries

Baked potato with broccoli and cheese, side salad, and fresh pineapple slices

Roast beef or ham sandwich, cup of tomato soup, and some grapes

Peanut butter and jelly sandwich, bowl of vegetable soup, and an apple

DINNER IDEAS IN THE CAMPUS DINING HALL

CHOOSE MORE OFTEN

Veggie-burger on a bun, salad, and fresh fruit

Chicken burrito with salsa and a side of vegetables, topped off with an orange

Grilled chicken breast, mashed potatoes, and carrots with two cookies and a light hot cocoa

Vegetable pizza, side salad, and fresh fruit

Pasta with vegetables and tomato sauce, sprinkled with parmesan cheese, and some Jell-O

Broiled fish with sautéed vegetables over rice and a frozen yogurt cone with sprinkles

Vegetarian chili, a large salad, and some angel food cake

Chicken kabob, veggies over rice, topped off with a frozen yogurt banana spilt

Large salad with beans, bowl of minestrone soup, and fruit ices

Lightly stir-fried shrimp and vegetables over linguini with sliced peaches for dessert

Chicken fajitas with salsa and a frozen fruit bar

The Infamous "Freshman Fifteen"

College is the time to gain knowledge—*not weight*. So why do so many freshman girls (and some guys), put on the pounds during their first year of school?

You can partially blame it on a decline in your RMR (Resting Metabolic Rate, also known as Basal Metabolic Rate, is the number of calories that you burn when your body is not active). Most little kids have super high RMR's—they can eat a ton, and not gain any weight. But, as you age and enter adulthood, your RMR usually slows down and you can't burn calories so effortlessly anymore. (At least that's true for the majority of us. Some people maintain wicked high metabolisms forever and ever, lucky devils.)

The undeniable reason for the increased weight (better known as the notorious "freshman fifteen" pounds of flub) is poor eating habits and lack of exercise. Let's take a look at some of the common culprits.

Late Night Munchies and Ordering In

Many college students make a habit of skipping meals, only to find themselves ravenous late at night. Does this sound familiar: "Hello Domino's, I'd like to order a large supreme pizza." Your body needs fuel *throughout* the day, not at the end of your day (like when you eat that family size bag of Doritos at 2 A.M.). Keep in mind: Calories eaten during the day are much more likely to be burned than calories eaten just before bedtime (unless your an extraordinarily active sleepwalker) because you burn more calories while active than while laying around. Take advantage of the campus dining hall during regular mealtimes and avoid the unnecessary eating late at night.

Vending Machines

STOP! Don't push that button before you've inspected the goods. Tragically enough, the majority of tempting treats that scream out "Eat me! Eat me!" from behind the glass windows are loaded with fat. For example, a bag of M&M's has 10 grams of fat, a Snickers bar has 14 grams of fat, two jumbo chocolate chip cookies have 18 grams of fat, and those "only sold in vending machines" cheese and crackers contain 11 grams of fat. Remember, the object of a healthy eating plan is to take in less than 30% of your total calories from fat, and one of the vending machine losers can really dent your day.

What's worse, you can't escape them. These machines are conveniently located in the dorms, classroom buildings, and student unions (close your eyes, don't even look). As for the times that you absolutely can't pass by without sticking your change into the slot, shoot for the healthier alternatives. For instance, fresh fruit, pretzels, fig bars, low-fat granola bars, and wheat crackers. And if your sweet tooth won't let up, *occasionally* satisfy the junk-food urge with hard candies, licorice, jelly beans, gummy bears, and other gooey-chewies. They don't provide anything in the way of nutrition *(mucho sugar)* but at least they are generally low in fat (sort of the best of the worst).

Getting Sloppy in the Dining Hall

Piling your tray with unhealthy, high-fat foods during mealtimes can also make you a candidate for "Miss Hefty Hips USA"! (or, "Mr. Larger than Life Lovehandles"—don't want to discriminate against the guys). No more excuses, it's time for some major damage control. Learn the CHOOSE MORE OFTENs cold, in the section we discussed earlier titled "Making The Grade in the Campus Dining Hall."

Lack of Exercise

Another common weight gain culprit is inactivity. The name of the game is balance—calories in equals calories out. In other words, eating a lot of garbage and sitting around on your butt all day (whether studying or watching soap operas) will put on the pounds, simply because you are taking in more calories than you are burning off. All types of exercise burns calories, walking, jumping rope, aerobic classes, stair climbing—it doesn't necessarily have to be something intense.

Moral of the story: Avoid all the unnecessary eating when you are just bored and looking for something to do, and get out there and move. Don't forget to read the Chapters 13 and 14 on exercise.

Alcohol and Partying

It's true, some studies suggest that an occasional drink can actually benefit your health. But come on, who are we kidding, that's not the kind of drinking most college kids are into. It's more like PARTY ALL NIGHT AND DRINK TILL YOU DROP. Maybe I can convince you to ease up on the booze by first providing the caloric facts. Alcohol is loaded with calories. More specifically, it is loaded "nutrient-less" calories (seven per gram, to be exact). Just another possible reason for weight gain.

Alcoholic Beverage	Serving Size (fluid ounces)	Approximate Calories
Beer	12	150
Light Beer	12	100
Bloody Mary	5	115
Gin and Tonic	7.5	170
Daiquiri	4.5	250

continues

continued

Alcoholic Beverage	Serving Size (fluid ounces)	Approximate Calories
Piña Colada	4.5	260
Screwdriver	7	175
Tequila Sunrise	5.5	190
Tom Collins	7.5	120
Gin/Rum/Vodka/Whiskey 100 proof	1.5 (1 shot)	125
Gin/Rum/Vodka/Whiskey 80 proof	1.5 (1 shot)	100
Wine, red and white	5	105
Champagne	5	133
Martini	2.5	155

And incidentally, alcohol can also lead to late night eating. One of my clients Lisa, reminisces of a pizza place located right next door to the popular off-campus bar. Every Thursday, Friday, and Saturday night, the place would be mobbed with semi-drunk kids pigging out on pizza, all claiming "Purple Pizza" (the name of the place) had the best pizza in the entire world. Ironically enough, one day Lisa stopped in and had a slice for lunch without her usual alcohol buzz. Guess what? It wasn't even edible!

Whether you munch out with a group of friends, or devour your roommate's Pop-tart stash, alcohol can certainly cloud your thinking and instigate a late night eating orgy.

Another reason to lay off the booze: "Oh my aching head." You can literally lose an entire day between the headaches, nausea, fatigue, and other lousy symptoms that occur from drinking "one too many."

Alcohol Management 101: for the *occasional* times you drink:

➤ Make sure you have food in your stomach before you drink. Food can act as a buffer, and delay the absorption of alcohol into the bloodstream.

➤ Know your limit. Everyone has their own capacity for alcohol, and it's important to know when to stop. Bear in mind that you will not impress a potential crush if you are vomiting all over yourself at a party.

➤ Ask the bartender to dilute your drinks with extra fruit juice, seltzer water, or club soda. Also order wine spritzers ($1/2$ wine–$1/2$ seltzer).

➤ Alternate every other drink at a party with plain water, fruit juice, or any other non-alcoholic beverage. This way you're never empty-handed.

➤ My own personal advice: stick with non-alcoholic drinks and avoid alcohol altogether.

POP QUIZ—Did You Really Pay Attention to the Chapter?

So you think you know everything there is to know about eating healthy on campus? Well strut your stuff by taking the following quiz. (The answers can be found on the next page.)

1. Circle the two beverages which are best bets in the campus dining hall:

   a. Sweetened iced teas
   b. Water
   c. Orange Juice
   d. Soda

2. Which one of the following sandwiches has the most fat?

   a. Tuna fish sandwich
   b. Roast beef sandwich
   c. Turkey breast sandwich
   d. Grilled chicken sandwich

3. Eating breakfast can help you control your weight?

   a. True
   b. False

4. A low-fat topping for a baked potato is:

   a. Sour cream
   b. Butter
   c. Margarine
   d. Marinara Sauce

5. Choose the breakfast cereal that offers the most fiber:

   a. Captain Crunch
   b. Raisin Bran
   c. Rice Krispies
   d. Frosted Flakes

6. Which type of potato has the most fat?

   a. Baked potato
   b. Roasted potato
   c. French- fried potato
   d. Mashed potato

7. Circle the following high-fat salad bar items:

   a. Olives
   b. Beans
   c. Bacon Bits
   d. Chick Peas

8. Which is the healthier soup?

   a. Cream of broccoli
   b. Vegetable Barley

9. It is perfectly okay to eat lean red meat once in awhile?

   a. True
   b. False

10. Some of the healthiest desserts found in the campus dining hall include:

    a. Applesauce
    b. Frozen yogurt
    c. Angel food cake
    d. All of the above

Answers: 1) b and c 2) a 3) True 4) d 5) b 6) c 7) a and c 8) b 9) True 10) d

The Least You Need to Know

➤ Take responsibility for yourself and select well-balanced, healthy meals in the campus dining hall.

➤ Don't forget to start your day with a nutritious breakfast. Eating breakfast helps regulate your appetite throughout the rest of the day so you won't overeat during lunch and dinner.

➤ Avoid those dreaded "Freshman fifteen" pounds by dodging vending machines, stopping late night ordering in, making low-fat selections in the campus dining hall, and getting off the couch to exercise.

➤ Alcohol contains a lot of "empty calories," and excessive drinking may result in weight gain.

Part 7
Weight Management 101

Weight control seems to be a full time job for some people—on and off every diet on the planet! I have a friend, Joan, who once told me her biggest fear of death is that they will print her weight in the obituary! Needless to say, she's alive and well, and on another cockamamie diet fad.

It's finally time to stop going up and down like a yo-yo, and stick with a sensible plan of attack. Whether you want to lose weight, gain weight, or most importantly, stop obsessing, this final section covers it all, so read on. I'll provide weight loss programs to help knock off (and keep off) those extra unwanted pounds, along with calorie-cramming strategies to help you skinny folks beef up your bods. I'll also take a look at life-threatening eating disorders, and where to find help when food and exercise go beyond health and get way out of control.

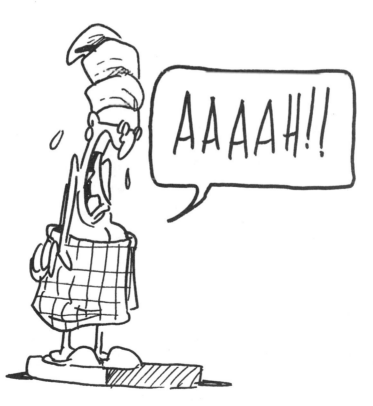

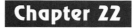

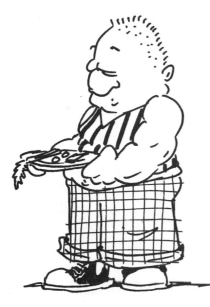

Chapter 22

Come On, Knock It Off

In This Chapter

➤ Why crash dieting *doesn't* work

➤ Identifying your ideal body weight

➤ Lose weight on a well-balanced program

➤ Understanding the language of "bubbles"

➤ Maintaining a healthy body weight forever

Let's take a walk down memory lane. We've had the Scarsdale diet, the grapefruit diet, the banana-cottage cheese diet, the cabbage soup diet, the *no* carbohydrate diet, and even the "lose 10 pounds in a week by eating just popcorn and mashed potatoes diet" (obviously written by a very constipated psychopath).

Unfortunately, crash dieting has always been (and remains to be) an American sport that just won't go away, sort of like trick candles on a birthday cake, each time you blow one out another pops right up to taunt you. But the jokes on us. With all of these blubber blasting gimmicks, our national waistline continues to bulge! In fact, most people that lose weight on these wacko programs wind up gaining it all back—*plus* some extra pounds to boot! This is commonly known as the yo-yo effect. What's more, the fad diets usually leave you deprived and irritable.

So, What's the Best Diet Anyway?

If you're looking for a quick fix, close the book. This chapter is *not* going to help you. The bottom line is that people should lose weight eating the very same healthy foods that they will continue to eat *after* they have lost the weight. That is, lots of complex carbs coming from whole grains, fruits and vegetables, low-fat dairy, and lean sources of protein foods. Makes perfect sense right? I mean, to lose weight *forever,* you must work on changing your eating behavior forever! Come on and give the bubble plan that I'm going to present to you later in this chapter, a try. You've got nothing to lose except your saggy saddlebags, bulging belly, flabby grandma arms (sorry grandma Martha), and size extra-large underwear.

Food for Thought

A sensible weight loss plan should shed pounds slow but steady (otherwise it's just a lot of water, *not* fat)—approximately one to two pounds per week, which works out to around four to eight pounds per month.

What Should You Weigh? Identifying Your Ideal Body Weight

First things first, figure out a realistic weight to strive for. The most commonly used measure for determining a healthy weight has been the Metropolitan Life Insurance Company's Height/Weight Tables, which were established and based on the ratios of insured people with the greatest longevity. While this table is a valuable tool, it should only be used as a general guideline because it covers a broad range of numbers for each height category.

First find out what size frame you are:

TO APPROXIMATE YOUR FRAME SIZE

Bend forearm upward at a 90 degree angle. Keep fingers straight and turn the inside of your wrist toward your body. Place thumb and index finger of other hand on the two prominent bones on either side of the elbow. Measure space between your fingers on a ruler. (A physician would use a caliper.) Compare with tables below listing elbow measurements for medium-framed men and women. Measurements lower than those listed indicate small frame. Higher measurements indicate large frame.

Men Height	Elbow Breadth	Women Height	Elbow Breadth
5' 1" - 5' 2"	2 1/2" - 2 7/8"	4' 9" - 5' 2"	2 1/4" - 2 1/2"
5' 3" - 5' 6"	2 5/8" - 2 7/8"	5' 3" - 5' 10"	2 3/8" - 2 5/8"
5' 7" - 5' 10"	2 3/4" - 3"	5' 11"	2 1/2" - 2 3/4"
5' 11" - 6' 2"	2 3/4" - 3 1/8"		
6' 3"	2 7/8" - 3 1/4"		

Used with permission of the Metropolitan Life Insurance Companies. Heights taken without shoes.

MET LIFE HEIGHT AND WEIGHT TABLES No Shoes / No Clothes							
MEN age 25 and over				**WOMEN age 25 and over**			
Height Feet Inches	Small Frame	Medium Frame	Large Frame	Height Feet Inches	Small Frame	Medium Frame	Large Frame
5 1	123-129	126-136	133-145	4 9	99-108	106-118	115-128
5 2	125-131	128-138	135-148	4 10	100-110	108-120	117-131
5 3	127-133	130-140	137-151	4 11	101-112	110-123	119-134
5 4	129-135	132-143	139-155	5 0	103-115	112-126	122-137
5 5	131-137	134-146	141-159	5 1	105-118	115-129	125-140
5 6	133-140	137-149	144-163	5 2	108-121	118-132	128-144
5 7	135-143	140-152	147-167	5 3	111-124	121-135	131-148
5 8	137-146	143-155	150-171	5 4	114-127	124-138	134-152
5 9	139-149	146-158	153-175	5 5	117-130	127-141	137-156
5 10	141-152	149-161	156-179	5 6	120-133	130-144	140-160
5 11	144-155	152-165	159-183	5 7	123-136	133-147	143-164
6 0	147-159	155-169	163-187	5 8	126-139	136-150	146-167
6 1	150-163	159-173	167-192	5 9	129-142	139-153	149-170
6 2	153-167	162-177	171-197	5 10	132-145	142-156	152-173
6 3	157-171	166-182	176-202	5 11	135-148	145-159	155-176

Source; Adapted and used with permission from the Metropolitan Life Insurance Company, 1983. Weights at ages 25-59 based on lowest mortality.

Testing Your Body Fat: Getting Pinched, Dunked, and Zapped

Where your weight indicates the sum total of *all* your body parts, it doesn't take into consideration your body composition (the amount of body fat versus lean body mass), which is important to know since muscle weighs more than fat! In fact, some people may appear a bit high on the weight chart *but* have very little body fat, indicating that the weight is coming from muscle mass and *not* blubber mass.

To get a more accurate idea as to where you stand in terms of fat, checkout your body fat percentage by getting pinched, dunked, or zapped—especially if you regularly workout. Compare your results with the normative ranges in the chart below.

% Body Fat for Women		
AGE	GOOD	EXCELLENT
20-29	20.6 - 22.7	17.1 - 19.8
30-39	21.6 - 24.0	18.0 - 20.8
40-49	24.9 - 27.3	21.3 - 24.9
50-59	28.5 - 30.8	25.0 - 27.4
60+	29.3 - 31.8	25.1 - 28.5

% Body Fat for Men		
AGE	GOOD	EXCELLENT
20-29	14.1 - 16.8	9.4 - 12.9
30-39	17.5 - 19.7	13.9 - 16.6
40-49	19.6 - 21.8	16.3 - 18.8
50-59	21.3 - 23.4	17.9 - 20.6
60+	22.0 - 24.3	18.4 - 21.1

Skin-Fold Calipers

Getting "pinched" utilizes what are called *calipers*, a contraption that looks like a hand-gun with salad tongs. A tester positions the gun on certain parts of your body and grabs your fat so that it is pulled away from your muscle and bone. (Sounds painful, but it's actually not!) After gathering a few different measurements, typically from the back of your arm, your thigh, your abdomen, your shoulder, and your hip, the tester will plug each number into a formula to calibrate your overall body fat percentage.

Although the calipers are quick, simple, and convenient, the test results can sometimes be skewed if a tester pinches some muscle along with the fat *or* does not pinch enough of the fat. You will also need to have this type of test performed *before* a workout, during exercise your skin slightly swells which can make you appear fatter than you are. Yikes!

Food for Thought
Take a trained athlete and a couch potato of the same height and weight, the athlete looks healthier, leaner, and most likely wears a smaller clothing size than the couch spud. This is because muscle weighs more than fat, even though it takes up less space!

Food for Thought
Where do carry your excess padding, on your belly or butt? Studies have shown that people carrying excess fat on the upper body and stomach suffer *more* health risks than people carrying fat on the hips and buttocks.

Underwater Weighing

Getting "dunked" is actually the most accurate of the classic methods of body fat testing. Basically you sit on a scale that is situated in a small pool of warm water. Next, you blow *all* the air out of your lungs and dunk underneath until you are completely submerged for about five seconds. Your underwater weight will then register on a digital scale and be plugged into a formula to determine the percent of body fat.

Bio-Electrical Impedance

Getting "zapped" requires you to lie on your back with one electrode attached to your hand and another to your foot. A signal is then sent from one electrode to the other. The faster the signal travels, the more muscle you have. On the other hand, the slower the signal moves, the more fat you have because fat will impede or block the signal.

How Many Calories Should You Eat for Weight Loss and Weight Maintenance?

Counting the calories in each morsel of food that you eat is *not* the way to go. But you can get a general idea of how many total calories you should eat each day, to either maintain *or* lose weight, with the following formula.

1. First find your BMR (that's your Basal Metabolic Rate *or* the amount of calories needed to perform your normal bodily functions at rest).

   BMR = your current weight × 10

2. Next, multiply your BMR × an activity factor

   BMR × 0.30 (for average daily activities)

3. Last, add your BMR + activity factor together

Here's an example of a 130-pound woman;

   130 pounds × 10 = BMR of 1,300 calories

   1,300 calories × .30 = 390 activity factor

   1,300 + 390 = 1,690 calories per day

People who participate in regular physical activity more than four times a week will need to raise the activity factor to .40–.60.

The example above shows that an average 130-pound woman can maintain her weight on 1,690 calories per day. Now let's say she wanted to lose a few pounds. To *lose* weight, she would need to create a negative balance by reducing the amount of daily "maintaining" calories *and* upping her exercise to burn even more calories! For instance, she would need to get on a 1,400 calorie food plan, *plus* working out aerobically 4–5 days per week. She'd have no problem shedding some weight safely and efficiently.

Plug your own stats into the formula and figure out what it will take calorically, to melt away those unwanted pounds. Understand that *no one* should ever go lower than 1,200 calories per day—you will

> **Food for Thought**
> People are different, and will lose weight at different speeds on different plans. For instance, you and your friend may do the math and come up with the same 1,400 calorie weight loss plan, but when you both begin the program she may lose 1–2 pounds each week, and you may only lose $1/2$ pound each week. In this case, assume that you have a slower metabolism and need to step up your exercise and go to the lower 1,200 calorie plan.

slow down your metabolism *and* set yourself up to gain all the weight back. Even if you are very petite, and the math works out to be less than 1,200—stick with 1,200 calories and jack up your exercise.

The "Bubble Game" and Your Personal Weight Loss Plan

Now that you've done the math, roll up your sleeves and get ready to select one of the following well-balanced, weight loss plans: 1,200 cals, 1,400 cals, 1,600 cals, or 1,800 cals, *or* play around and create an in-between plan of your own. Make it into a game and simply follow the bubble sheets by focusing on the number of total daily servings from each of the five food groups. Notice that all the calculations have been done for you, so there's no need to count a single calorie. In fact, calorie counting from here on in is off limits!

Understanding the Bubbles, What Counts as What?

So what the heck are all these bubbles? A bubble is simply a serving size, therefore, the amount of bubbles after each food group is the total amount of servings your plan has for each day. For example, if you are following the 1,200 calorie plan, you have two fruit bubbles and four grain/bread bubbles, meaning two servings of fruit and four servings of grain. Browse below at the various items under each food category, and learn exactly what counts as one serving so that you know how to plan out your foods for the day.

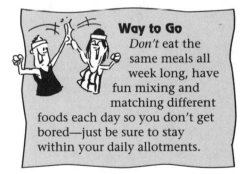

Way to Go
Don't eat the same meals all week long, have fun mixing and matching different foods each day so you don't get bored—just be sure to stay within your daily allotments.

It's *not* necessary to weigh or measure, an eyeball guesstimation will work just fine. Here's how to guesstimate your serving sizes, and remember, this is only a general list—there are a gazillion other foods that can fit perfectly into each category, so go ahead and plug in your favorites.

One Grain/Bread Bubble =

1 medium slice of *any* type of bread

$^1/_2$ small bagel or English muffin

small pita bread

1 serving cereal (hot or cold)

$^1/_2$ cup cooked pasta, rice, barley or cous-cous

small baked potato or sweet potato (size of your closed fist)

$^1/_2$ cup peas or corn

1 ounce (small bag) pretzels

low-fat granola bar

2 fig cookies

*Note: Some vegetables are included in this group because they are very starchy.

**Here's some common grains and how they can count

pasta entree = four grain bubbles

side of pasta or rice = two grain bubbles

large baked potato = two grain bubbles

large, hot pretzel = three grain bubbles

potato knish = three grain bubbles

large New York bagel = three to four grain bubbles

One Vegetable Bubble = (most vegetables are unlimited, just make sure to eat your *minimal* quota!)

1 cup raw vegetables

$^1/_2$ cup cooked vegetables

1 cup vegetable juice

**the only exceptions are the starchy potatoes, peas, and corn, which get counted as grain.

One Fruit Bubble =

any medium size piece of fruit (apple, banana, pear, etc.)

$^1/_2$ small cantaloupe

large wedge of watermelon or honey dew

1 cup fresh fruit salad or berries

small glass fruit juice (about $^1/_2$ cup)

large scoop of fruit sorbet

frozen fruit bar

small handful of dried fruit

One Milk Bubble =

1 cup low-fat milk (skim or 1%)

1 8-ounce container of nonfat (flavored) yogurt

small low-fat frozen yogurt

3 slices of low-fat hard cheese (*or* 1 $^1/_2$ ounces)

$^3/_4$ cup (big scoop) low-fat cottage cheese

1 cup low-fat pudding

skim milk; cappuccino, café latté, or hot cocoa

4 Tablespoons parmesan cheese

1 Milk *plus* 1 Fat =

1 cup whole milk

regular cheese on anything

one scoop real ice cream

regular hot chocolate, cappuccino, or café latté

1 cup chocolate pudding

anything else made with whole milk

One Protein Bubble = approximately three ounces of lean meat, poultry, or fish (the size of a deck of cards), unless otherwise indicated.

chicken breast (3 ounces)

turkey breast (3 ounces)

lean red meats (3 ounces)

turkey burger or veggie burger (3 ounces)

all seafood and fish (3 ounces)

tofu ($^2/_3$ cup)

egg whites (approximately 4)

whole eggs (2)

beans ($^1/_2$ –1 cup cooked)

One Fat Bubble =

*anytime you *think* something is prepared with fat, or

*anytime you use; 1 teaspoon butter, oil, margarine, or mayonnaise

*1 Tablespoon cream cheese, peanut butter, or salad dressing

*2 Tablespoons of sour cream

For reduced-calorie spreads double the serving size, and you do *not* need to count fat-free spreads at all.

At last, the "Free Foods" that don't count as anything!

Mustard	Cocktail sauce
Ketchup	Salsa
*Soy sauce	Tomato sauce
*Teriyaki sauce	*Bouillon
Worcester sauce	Sugar
All spices and seasonings	Sugar substitutes
Jams and jellies	Hard candies (3 per day)
Pancake syrup (a figure 8 only)	Chewing gum (1 pack per day)
Fat-free salad dressings and spreads	Coffee/tea
Horseradish	Sugar-free beverages

*these foods are extremely high in salt, when available choose the low-sodium versions.

Tracking Your Food on the Daily Bubble Sheets

Make 20-plus Xerox copies of the food-plan that's right for you and chart your daily food intake for the first few weeks, just to get the hang of it. After eating each meal or snack, cross off the appropriate bubbles at the bottom. This will help you to keep an accurate eye on exactly how much food you've already eaten, *and* how much is left for the rest of the day.

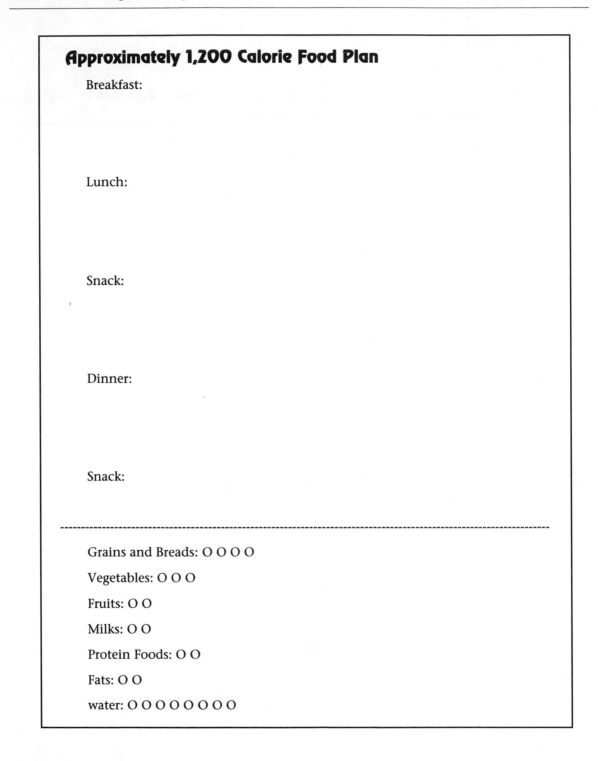

Approximately 1,200 Calorie Food Plan

Breakfast:

Lunch:

Snack:

Dinner:

Snack:

- -

Grains and Breads: O O O O

Vegetables: O O O

Fruits: O O

Milks: O O

Protein Foods: O O

Fats: O O

water: O O O O O O O O

Ready Made Menu

Sample day of 1,200 calorie food plan

Breakfast: 1 serving of cereal
1 cup skim milk
$^1/_2$ small cantaloupe

Lunch: large salad with 3 ounces grilled chicken with
2 tablespoons low-fat Italian salad dressing
small pita bread

Snack: small frozen yogurt

Dinner: 3 ounces of grilled shrimp in lemon
lots of steamed broccoli
large baked potato
with 1 teaspoon of margarine
1 cup fresh strawberries

Grains O O O O

Vegetables O O O

Fruit O O

Milk O O

Protein O O

Fat O O

Water O O O O O O O O

Approximately 1,400 Calorie Food Plan

Breakfast:

Lunch:

Snack:

Dinner:

Snack:

Grains and Breads: O O O O O

Vegetables: O O O

Fruits: O O O

Milks: O O

Protein Foods: O O

Fats: O O

water: O O O O O O O O

Ready Made Menu

Sample day of 1,400 food calorie plan

Breakfast: toasted English muffin with
1 tablespoon cream cheese
1 cup skim milk *plus* 1 cup blueberries in a blender with ice

Lunch: 3 ounces turkey breast
2 slices whole wheat bread
lettuce, tomato slices, and mustard
apple

Snack: an orange

Dinner: tossed green salad with fat-free dressing
3 ounces grilled fish in lemon
small baked potato with 2 Tablespoons sour cream
steamed spinach with 2–4 Tablespoons parmesan cheese

Grains O O O O O

Vegetables O O O O

Fruits O O O

Milks O O

Protein O O

Fats O O O

Water O O O O O O O O

Approximately 1,600 Calorie Food Plan

Breakfast:

Lunch:

Snack:

Dinner:

Snack:

- -

Grains and Breads: O O O O O O

Vegetables: O O O

Fruits: O O O

Milk: O O O

Protein Foods: O O

Fats: O O O

Water: O O O O O O O O

Ready Made Menu

Sample day of 1,600 calorie food plan

Breakfast: bowl of oatmeal with skim milk
container of nonfat flavored yogurt
small glass orange juice

Lunch: turkey burger on bun
side salad with 1 tablespoon dressing
fresh fruit salad

Snack: low-fat granola bar or
frozen fruit bar

Dinner: stir-fry chicken and *lots* of veggies (use only 1–2 teaspoons oil and soy sauce)
1 cup brown rice
small frozen yogurt

Grains and Breads: O O O O O O

Vegetables: O O O O O

Fruits: O O O

Milk: O O O

Protein Foods: O O

Fats: O O O

Water: O O O O O O O O

Approximately 1,800 Calorie Food Plan

Breakfast:

Lunch:

Snack:

Dinner:

Snack:

Grains and Breads: O O O O O O O

Vegetables: O O O O O O

Fruits: O O O O

Milk: O O O

Protein Foods: O O

Fats: O O O

Water: O O O O O O O O

Ready Made Menu

Sample day of 1,800 calorie food plan

Breakfast: egg white omelet with veggies (use nonstick cooking spray)
2 slices whole wheat toast with 2 teaspoons reduced-fat margarine
sliced bananas and strawberries (~1 cup)
1 cup of skim milk

Lunch: 1 slice vegetable cheese pizza
frozen fruit pop

Snack: peach
2 fig cookies

Dinner: grilled swordfish (~3 ounces),
marinate in lemon and 1 tsp. olive oil
1 cup pasta with marinara sauce
grated skim milk mozzarella cheese (1 1/2 oz)
cooked carrots and green beans
a baked apple

Grains and Breads: O O O O O O O

Vegetables: O O O O O O

Fruits: O O O O

Milk: O O O

Protein Foods: O O

Fats: O O O

Water: O O O O O O O O

No More "I've Blown It" Syndrome, All Foods Are Allowed

Are you guilty of the "all-or nothing" mentality? Do you place all your faves "off-limits" when you are dieting, and the second you eat anything on the "bad list," you go whole hog and eat the house? ("I've already blown it—may as well polish off the rest of the chips and cookies. I'll start fresh on Monday.")

Diets can fail when you are deprived of your favorite foods—even if they aren't so healthy. You *don't* gain weight from occasionally eating moderate amounts of high-fat foods. In fact, you *lose* weight because in the end you don't feel deprived, and are able to continue on your weight loss program.

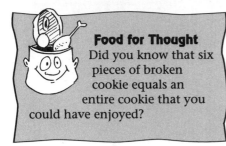

Food for Thought
Did you know that six pieces of broken cookie equals an entire cookie that you could have enjoyed?

The following list shows you that almost *anything* can fit in, you'll just have to cross off the appropriate bubbles and account for the food item during that day. Of course, try your best to stick with healthier choices most of the time, but go ahead and occasionally splurge on pizza, cookies, cake, and anything else that tempts your palate—I encourage it! Simply stay within your daily bubble limit by shifting other meals around to compensate, and you'll still lose weight!

Fat-Combo Foods

Cookies (2 medium) = 1 grain, 1 fat

Cake (medium slice, *any* type) = 2 grains, 2 fats

Doughnut = 2 grains, 2 fats

Large bakery cookie = 2 grains, 2 fats

Scone (medium) = 2 grains, 2 fats

Danish/pastry = 2 grains, 2 fats

Bakery muffin (large) = 3 grains, 2 fats

Potato chips (small bag) = 1 grain, 1 fat

Corn chips (small bag) = 1 grain, 1 fat

Chocolate bar (Kit-Kat, Snickers, and so on) = 1 grain, 3 fats

Coleslaw ($^1/_2$ cup) = 1 vegetable, 1 fat

Potato salad ($^1/_2$ cup)= 1 grain, 1 fat

Real ice cream (2 scoops) = 2 milks, 2 fats

French fries (about 20) = 2 grains, 2 fats

Chinese Lomein (1 cup) = 2 grains, 2 fats

Cornbread (medium piece) = 1 grain, 1 fat

Cream soups (1 cup) = 1 grain, 1 fat, 1 vegetable

Macaroni and cheese (1 cup) = 2 grains, 1 milk or protein), 1 fat

Pizza (1 medium slice) = 2 grains, 1 milk or protein), 1 fat

**notice that for macaroni and cheese and pizza, the cheese can either be counted as milk *or* protein.

276

Setting Realistic Goals

Don't get yourself overwhelmed with a tremendous amount of weight that you need to lose. Instead, break it into smaller, more achievable short-term goals. For example, if you have your heart set on losing, say, 40 pounds, aim for 10 pounds at a time. Even with a mere eight pounds to lose, strive for knocking off two pounds at a time.

Also, understand that genetics plays a *key* role in determining your body makeup, so don't dream about that "barbie-doll body" because it's not gonna happen. Take a look at your mom, dad, and other relatives, although, biology isn't destiny, heredity does play an integral part in shaping your shape.

The most important thing is to learn to love the body you have and keep your focus on ways to make it healthy. You may never be a size six or have bulging muscles, but you can learn to be happy with the body you have when you take care of it.

Don't Obsess Over the Scale, It Can Drive You Nuts!

Don't let the normal day-to-day fluctuations due to water, salt, and hormones throw you into a state of panic. Limit the amount of times you weigh yourself to no more than once or twice a week. In fact, avoid hopping on the scale each time you hit the bathroom by packing it away in the closet between weigh-ins, *or* simply weigh yourself outside your home (at the gym, your doctor's office, and so on).

Get Moving and Keep Moving

Following a healthy food plan is only half the weight loss equation—you gotta move to lose!! Numerous studies have shown that exercise helps promote weight loss *and* weight maintenance by revving up your metabolism (that is, burning more calories). What's more, exercise relieves stress, *and* can even psych up your state of mind so that you're motivated to make smart food choices during the day. Flip back to Chapters 13 and 14 and memorize!

Maintaining Your Weight After You've Lost It

So you have reached your goal—now what? HOORAY on one hand, EEK on the other! Maintaining your weight is actually *harder* than losing weight because there's no number goal to strive for, you're already there. Hang tight and read the following tips, this time your shapely physique is here to stay.

➤ The trick is to loosen the diet reins, but not too much. Continue with a *modified* version of your bubble plan (in your head only), since it's super well-balanced and encourages you to eat healthfully.

➤ Figure out a five-pound weight range with your present weight in the middle. For example, if your weight is 130 pounds give yourself a range of 128–132 pounds. Continue to weigh-in once a week, and if you go over the range get back on the bubble sheets.

Food for Thought

If you decide to work with a nutritionist, remember, you want a food partner, *not* a food fanatic dictator! Be sure to find a qualified Registered Dietitian (RD) that will go at your pace and make you feel completely comfortable. For a registered dietitian in your area, call the American Dietetic Association at 1-800-366-1655.

➤ Plan one "meal off" each week. In other words, a meal that doesn't fit or calculate into your plan (anything you'd like). If your weight continues to stay put, add in a second "meal off" or possibly a dessert. Play around and see what your body can handle, everyone is different.

➤ You may prefer to simply add a few more grains to your plan (*or* a fruit and milk). See what your weekly weigh-ins reveal and never panic if it slightly shifts upward. Simply take away some of the additions the following week. Remember, the key to maintaining is to find out how much food your body can handle.

➤ Absolutely continue with your regular exercise program. Exercise allows you to eat more food since it burns mega calories, *and* keeps you tight and toned since it zaps body fat and increases your lean body mass!

The Least You Need to Know

➤ Fad diets don't work. People should lose weight eating the very same healthy foods they will continue to eat after the weight is lost.

➤ A popular table for finding your ideal body weight is the Metropolitan Life Insurance Height/Weight Table.

➤ Your weight on the scale is the sum total of *all* your body parts (fat mass and lean mass), therefore, it's also helpful to test your *body fat percentage* since this specifically identifies how much of your body is actually fat.

➤ Don't set your heart on a Barbie/Ken-doll body—that's just not going to happen. Plan realistic weight loss goals by understanding that genetics plays a *key* role in body make-up.

➤ Learn to love the body you have, and focus on making it healthy, not necessarily model shaped.

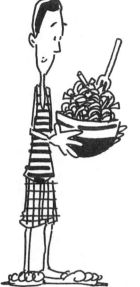

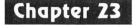

Chapter 23

Say You Wanna Put on a Few Pounds?

In This Chapter

➤ Strategies to help you gain weight

➤ High-calorie meals and snacks

➤ Refreshing shakes to boost your calories

Is your metabolism so speedy that you burn calories quicker than you can pack 'em in? Maybe you're one of those "uninterested in food" people who looks down at your watch and thinks "Oops, I forgot to eat lunch." Whatever the reasons behind your thin body, fear not, with some effort and determination you can start an upward trend on your bathroom scale.

Six Tips to Help You Pack in the Calories

Gaining weight requires devouring *more* calories than you burn. Stick with the basic food principles and concentrate on the following tips:

➤ Eat larger portions at your three main meals—even consider adding an extra meal to your day.

➤ Snacks are mega important! Plan at least three snacks a day. Snack number 1 can fit between breakfast and lunch; snack number 2, between lunch and dinner; snack number 3 before bedtime. Tote along in your bag trail-mix, dried fruits, crackers, fig bars, and nuts. Also keep them in your desk at work.

➤ Add calorically dense foods to your meals. For example, toss beans, seeds, nuts, peas, avocado, cheese, and dressings into salads. Add shrimp, fish, chunks of chicken, and lots of parmesan cheese to pastas. Add crackers, rice, corn, noodles, and beans to your soups. And don't forget about the bread basket; spread on the margarine and dig in!

➤ Guzzle tons of pure fruit juice or milk (preferably not skim, but not whole either) with and between your meals; it's a great way to painlessly add calories.

➤ Try some of the calorically dense supplements such as Ensure Plus™, Sustacal™, Boost™, Carnation Instant Breakfast™, and Nutriment™. Just make sure you drink them *between* meals or *with* meals, not instead of meals, or you'll defeat the whole purpose of extra calories.

➤ Consult a qualified exercise trainer about embarking on a weight lifting program. It can build up your muscle *plus* put on some pounds.

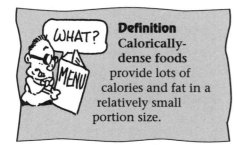

Definition
Calorically-dense foods provide lots of calories and fat in a relatively small portion size.

Although, the idea is to increase your calories, you also want to keep your diet well-balanced and nutritious. Don't shovel in chocolate bars, donuts, cakes, cookies, and other "nutrient-less" stuff that will slam you with fat and supply zippo in the nutrition department. Instead, stick with foods that are calorically dense, *and* provide lots of nutrients at the same time. Here are some examples:

Start with a Basic, Healthy Meal	To Add Some Calories
Vegetable Omelet	Add cheese and a bagel with margarine
Salads	Add shredded cheese, avocado, olives, and plenty of dressing
Pizza	Add extra cheese and vegetables
Pasta	Add olive oil and parmesan cheese
Chicken Stir-fry	Add peanuts or cashews
Burritos	Add guacamole or sour cream

High-Calorie Snack Ideas

frozen yogurt milkshake (anything goes)

tortilla chips with salsa and guacamole

bran, corn, or blueberry muffins

cheese and crackers

dried fruit and nut mixture

bowl of cereal with fruit and low-fat milk

peanut butter and jelly on crackers

peanut butter on apple slices or bananas

cereal mixed with yogurt

fruit bars and granola bars

Shake It Up Baby

Shakes can be a refreshing, filling alternative to snacks, and can add a significant amount of calories to your day.

Try these ideas:

1. Process in a blender: 4 ice cubes, $\frac{1}{2}$ cup orange juice, $\frac{1}{2}$ cup of melon chunks, 1 banana or $\frac{1}{2}$ cup strawberries and wheat germ (optional). Add more or less juice/fruit to achieve the desired consistency.

2. Mix Carnation Instant Breakfast™ or Ovaltine™ with 1 cup of low-fat milk—drink it *with* your breakfast, or have it for a midmorning or bedtime snack.

3. Purée 10 oz. silken tofu, $\frac{3}{4}$ cup apple juice, 1 banana, or $\frac{1}{2}$ cup blueberries in a blender and top with walnuts or almonds.

4. For a thick smoothy, purée 1 cup yogurt, 2 teaspoons honey, 1 banana, and $\frac{3}{4}$ cup fruit juice (pineapple or orange juice works well). Mix in wheat germ if desired.

MENU

Ready Made Menu

Wanna gain some weight? Try this sample menu:

Breakfast
bran flakes (large bowl)
low-fat milk
2 handfuls of raisins
large glass of orange juice
bagel with margarine

continues

continued

snack 1
8 oz. low-fat milk *with* Carnation Instant Breakfast™
large blueberry muffin

Lunch

chicken salad sandwich on whole wheat bread
bowl of vegetable soup with crackers
apple
large glass of fruit juice

snack 2
peanut butter on crackers with low-fat milk
dried fruit and nuts
glass of juice

Dinner:
vegetable cheese pizza
lots of Italian bread
salad with olive oil and vinegar
flavored fruit drink

Bedtime snack
frozen yogurt cone with sprinkles

The Least You Need to Know

➤ To gain weight you must take in *more* calories than your body burns.

➤ Increase your daily calories by eating bigger portions with your meals and by snacking on calorically-dense foods that also offer nutrition.

➤ Guzzle tons of fruit juice, make creative shakes, or drink the popular supplements that are on the market.

➤ Embark in a weight lifting program. It can help beef up your muscles and your weight.

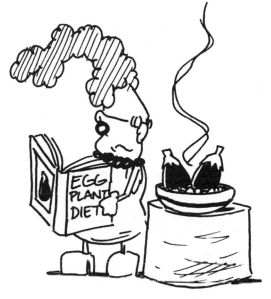

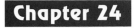

Understanding Eating Disorders

The ideal of beauty has become more and more slender, a bone-thin slender, in fact, that most people are *not* capable of achieving through healthy, normal eating. Deluged by skinnie-minnies from TV, movies, and magazines, it's no wonder that millions of Americans each year suffer from serious eating disorders. In fact, more than 90% of those afflicted with eating disorders are adolescents and young adult women, who are at a time in their life where the quest for that "ideal bod" is overwhelming.

Many psychological theories about eating disorders have been proposed and fortunately, today there are numerous comprehensive treatment centers to help people struggling with anorexia nervosa, bulimia, and compulsive overeating. As a society we need to overcome this obsession with *unreasonably* low weights and learn to accept and love the healthy genetic shapes we were given. This chapter provides you with the basics on eating disorders so that you can better understand the world of dieting gone haywire, and perhaps help a friend, a relative, or even yourself.

Anorexia Nervosa: The Relentless Pursuit of Thinness

Anorexia nervosa is a complex psychological disorder that literally involves self-induced starvation. People who suffer from this illness eat next to nothing, refuse to maintain a healthy body weight for their corresponding height, and frequently claim to "feel fat," even though they are obviously emaciated. Because anorexics are severely malnourished, they often experience the following symptoms of starvation: brittle nails and hair; dry skin; extreme sensitivity to the cold; anemia (low iron); lanugo (fine hair growth on body surface); loss of bone; swollen joints; and *dangerously* low blood pressure, heart rates, and potassium levels. If not caught and treated in time, victims of anorexia nervosa can literally "diet themselves to death."

The prevalence of anorexia nervosa is estimated at 0.1–0.6% of the general population, with 90% of the sufferers women, and roughly six percent boys and young men. Although any personality can fall victim to this life-threatening illness, most anorexics tend to be perfectionists who keep their feelings bottled up inside; straight-A students, good athletes, and citizens who always do the right thing. For anorexics, restricting and controlling food becomes a way to cope with just about anything.

Warning Signs of Anorexia Nervosa

➤ Abnormal weight loss of 15% (or more) of normal body weight with no known medical illness accounting for the loss. It can also be a failure to gain an expected amount of weight during a period of growth for younger children and adolescents.

➤ An intense fear of becoming fat or gaining weight, along with strict dieting and severe caloric restriction—despite a rail-thin appearance.

➤ In females, absence of at least three consecutive menstrual cycles otherwise expected to be normal.

➤ Always moving the diet "finish line" (i.e., just five more pounds and then I'll stop).

➤ Constant preoccupation with food. Anorexics will often cook and prepare food for others, while refusing to eat anything themselves.

➤ Distorted body image. For example, claiming to "have fat hips" despite the fact that scales and mirrors show that they are severely emaciated.

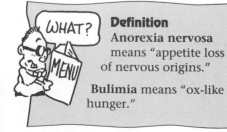

Definition
Anorexia nervosa means "appetite loss of nervous origins."

Bulimia means "ox-like hunger."

➤ Strange eating rituals such as cutting food up into tiny pieces, taking unusually long periods of time to eat a meal, *and* constantly preferring to eat alone.

➤ Obsessively over-exercising despite fatigue and weakness.

➤ Becoming socially withdrawn, isolated, and depressed.

A very special thanks to three of my clients who have allowed me to share their struggles with food.

"Weighting To Be Normal"

At 13 years of age, and 172 pounds, I wasn't very involved in the world around me. Sure, I saw the fried chicken, mashed potatoes, cakes, and cookies, but boys, clothing, and beaches alluded me. Don't get me wrong, I wasn't miserable all the time, I just wasn't particularly happy. In fact, most of the time I was nothing—I was just FAT!

Like most perfectionists, I seemed to do everything to extremes. Initially I ate to the fullest, and later when my doctor told me I needed to lose weight, I dieted to the skinniest! 365 days later and 52 pounds lighter, the new Jane emerged. I had exercised and dieted my way to health. Burgers and taxis were out, low-fat foods and biking were in!

Not surprisingly, my doctor was ecstatic with my success and my family was beaming with pride. My friends on the other hand, were filled with that strange combination of jealous admiration, and *finally* for the first time in my life, guys noticed me! They whistled when I walked down the street and approached me at school. "Wow," I thought. "If I can get this much attention at 120 pounds, imagine how great life could be at 110."

At 100 pounds I thought I had found bliss: I could count my ribs, pull down my pants without unbuttoning them, and most importantly, I could go an entire day on just a small fat-free frozen yogurt.

The months flew by, and my weight continued to plummet. Exhausted, freezing, and wearing size zero clothing, I had propelled myself into a lonely abyss. Summer nights felt like the dead of winter, and the urge to sleep was unstoppable. I knew I was sick—*everyone* knew I was sick—and I was ultimately diagnosed with anorexia nervosa.

Although I rejected the notion of having a disease, I struggled both mentally and physically with solid foods and decreasing my amount of exercise. *Gradually* over the course of a year I regained both my body and my life. I admit, low-fat foods and exercising are still entrenched in my life, but this time in a healthy manner, not as destructive disaster. I must push myself to eat a risky meal (a "scary" meal with fat) every other day, and allow myself to indulge in a dessert treat twice a week. Although I still obsess about my weight, it's no longer about losing; instead, it's about maintaining. I have been at my current *healthy* thin weight of 112 pounds for the last year and I guess you can say I have finally found an ideal way to exercise my "control." I "control" what I eat and how much I exercise, but this time not in a freezing abyss, rather, in a hot sweaty gym!

By Joan Stern, an 18-year-old recovered anorexic.

Bulimia Nervosa

The eating disorder termed bulimia is at least two or three times more prevalent than anorexia nervosa. In fact, recent surveys report about 1% of the general population, and 4% of women aged 18–30, suffer from this troublesome disease. People with bulimia have repeated episodes of *binge-eating*—rapidly consuming large quantities of food, and then ridding their bodies of the excess calories by vomiting, abusing laxatives or diuretics, or exercising obsessively. In most cases, this binge/purge syndrome is an outlet for anxiety, frustration, depression, loneliness, boredom, or sadness. Since most bulimics are typically normal weight, they can keep this a secret and go undetected for years. While some researchers think the problem is getting worse, others believe that people are just more willing to seek help, and therefore it's noticed and treated more often.

Warning Signs of Bulimia

Resources
For further reading, order

The Eating Disorder Catalog
Gurze Books, (800)-756-7533.

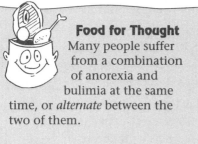

Food for Thought
Many people suffer from a combination of anorexia and bulimia at the same time, or *alternate* between the two of them.

Food for Thought
Eating disorders can sometimes run in families. In fact, the rate of anorexia among *sisters* has been estimated at 2–10%.

➤ Dissatisfaction with body shape and constant preoccupation with becoming thin.

➤ Recurrent mood swings and depression.

➤ Repeated episodes of rapidly consuming large amounts of food (binge-eating), followed by attempts to purge (get rid of food) through self-induced vomiting, use of laxatives or diuretics, prolonged exercise, or by following severe low-calorie diets in between binges.

➤ Serious physical complications from chronic vomiting, including erosion of dental enamel from acidic vomit, scars on the hands from sticking fingers down the throat, swollen glands, sore throat, irritation of the esophagus, and poor digestion (heartburn, gas, diarrhea, constipation, bloating). The more serious physical dangers include severe dehydration, loss of potassium (since potassium controls the heart beat), and rupture of the esophagus.

➤ Awareness that eating pattern is abnormal.

➤ Fear of not being able to control eating voluntarily.

➤ Light-headedness and dizziness or fainting.

➤ Frequent weight fluctuations of 10 pounds in either direction from the constant bingeing and purging.

"My Vicious Cycle of Starving-Stuffing"

It all started when I was preparing to go off to college. My anxiety stemmed from separating from my family and manifested itself in a body image and eating problem. Up until this time, I was a "normal" eater, eating when I was hungry, stopping when I was full, and occasionally overeating during special occasions. I ate chocolate bars, pizza, and movie theater popcorn without as much as a blink. What was it like then?

Suddenly, it was as if my body wasn't mine anymore. It became this "thing" separate from myself. I became hyper-aware and mentally obsessed with how to control my shape through obsessive exercise and restrictive eating patterns. Skipping two meals in a row and exercising two hours a day became normal to me. I used to stand in front of my dorm room mirror naked, poking and scrutinizing myself out loud. My self-esteem was so low that I actually needed someone to validate all of my insecurities. My overweight roommate would look on in disgust, reassuring me that I wasn't fat. A lot of people in my life got tired of reassuring me of this.

I did not allow myself to enjoy "forbidden foods" for a long time through college. I felt proud of this control, but ironically continued with my dissatisfaction over my "chunky body" (which has always been *very* thin, so I'm told). But after a while of rigid restriction, my body rebelled and my disordered eating took on a new twist: a few days of restricting (sometimes as low as 500 calories a day) and then bam—I would "sabotage" all of my efforts by stuffing myself until I was uncomfortably full! Feeling disgusted, depressed, and ENORMOUS, I would get rid of the calories by making myself vomit, and then struggle back to my extremely low-cal, restrictive diet, and the vicious cycle continued. My weight could fluctuate 10 pounds depending upon the day of the week, but to the outside world I still remained a "normal" little person.

I also developed strange idiosyncrasies. Certain colors had to be eaten together, and certain foods had to "match" each other for no particular reason, except for the fact that they made sense to me. I would also weigh myself up to 25 times each day. There was no room for error, spontaneity, or change.

Finally, coming to terms with the fact that this obsession with food and exercise was ruining my life, I started to see a psychotherapist. For the first time I realized that my "food thing" was only a symptom of unlimited emotions that I had bottled up inside. I needed to work hard to break free from my extremist attitudes and my belief that being less than perfect was not worth being (what is "perfect" anyway?).

Today, I allow myself to feel entitled to my words and actions, and realize that a middle ground is healthier in relation to feeling, thinking, and eating. I've also worked with a nutritionist for the past year. She has taught me that restricting inevitably leads to bingeing, and I'm desperately trying to do away with black/white days (restricting or bingeing), and instead focus on the "gray."

continues

continued

I no longer let one M&M dictate my self-esteem, and I have learned that normal eating is flexible and always changing. It's okay to eat a big piece of cake on my birthday, chocolate when I have PMS, and movie theater popcorn once in a while. "Normal eating" means eating healthy *most* of the time while allowing yourself to indulge when you feel like it. It's feeding yourself when you're hungry and sometimes when you are not—even just for the fun of it! It's feeding your mind as well as your body, and realizing that weight fluctuations are normal. It is seeing life as more than what you put in your mouth and enjoying social situations for the conversation and laughter. It is learning to accept our bodies, our strengths, and our limitations as well. I admit, everyday is a struggle right now, but at least I finally believe that I am worth it.

By a 26-year-old recovering bulimic.

Compulsive Overeating

Food for Thought
Many people aren't diagnosed with anorexia or bulimia, but suffer from less serious "food things" that nonetheless control and hinder their lives. Remember you only have one life to live. Get help and live it to the fullest!!

People who compulsively overeat repeatedly consume excessive amounts of food, sometimes to the point of abdominal discomfort. However, unlike bulimics, they do not get rid of the food with any of the methods mentioned above. In fact, most people with this type of eating disorder are overweight from the constant bingeing, and have a long history of weight fluctuations.

Since compulsive overeaters feel out of control with their food (and often eat in secret), there seems to be a high incidence of depression, in addition to the serious medical complications that go hand in hand with being overweight.

"Dieting My Way to Obesity"

The cycle began when I was 11 or 12. I wore a size 7 and thought I looked fat. I dieted, starved, exercised, overate, and ended up a size 9. I did the size 7–9 dance several times until I finally graduated to the 9–11 routine. This continued until I ultimately reached size 13.

The turning point from "eating problem" to "life-threatening disorder" happened in my adult years after the break-up of a serious relationship. I just couldn't face the anxiety of the dating world again! It was also right after my grandmother passed away and my father had a heart attack. Starting a high-powered, senior level job, my binges became out of control. Suddenly, walking home from work, I felt an urgent need to eat; I stopped at a grocery store, a deli, a restaurant, buying chips, cakes, ice cream, and cookies. I reached my apartment and rushed into the kitchen still wearing my heavy winter coat and hat, shoveling cake into my mouth. My hands were shaking, and not able to get the cake in fast enough! I finished the entire cake, a pint of ice cream, and 20 Oreos before I was finally calm enough to take off my coat and order Chinese take-out.

This routine went on night after night for months. Within six months I was up 85 pounds, and for the first time in my life, topped 200 pounds on the scale. I was depressed, desperate, and terrified. I cried on and off all day long—in the shower, on the train, and in my office, frantically searching for help from diet centers, obesity researchers, and hospital programs. I frequently and seriously contemplated suicide. I was humiliated and weighed 250 pounds. I felt like a heroin addict, only I was addicted to food.

With the understanding, support, and guidance from trusting, caring, and knowledgeable practitioners: a psychiatrist, a nutritionist, group therapy, *and* anti-depression medication, I am presently working my way out from this perpetual hell. I now follow a non-deprivational approach, *all* foods in moderation. Believe me, it took *a lot* for me to be willing to try this because all my life all I've ever known is either 750 calorie diets or 20,000 calorie binges. Today, I allow myself a chocolate bar if I really crave one, and if I need to overeat (not binge) because of a heavy stressful workload—I give myself permission.

I presently weigh 185 pounds, eat normally, and at 45, have a rebirth of hope.

By a 45-year-old compulsive overeater.

How to Help a Friend or Relative with an Eating Disorder

Combating an eating disorder is *huge* and generally involves a collaborative team of specialists including a *psychiatrist* (or psychologist) to work through the psychological dynamics, a *physician* to monitor physical status, and a *nutritionist* (or dietitian) to reintroduce food as an ally—not an enemy. Here are some of the things that you can do if you suspect a friend or family member has an eating disorder:

➤ Call your local hospital (or some of the treatment centers listed later in this chapter) and gather information on the various programs in your area. Ask about individual therapists, group therapy sessions, and nutritionists that specialize in food issues.

➤ In a very caring and gentle way, discuss your concerns with your friend or relative, and provide some of the professional resources and phone numbers that you've found. Be very supportive and patient—even offer to go along for any initial consults.

➤ If the person is a minor and refuses to get help, you may need to speak with a family member.

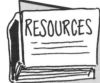

Resources

The following organizations can help provide information, literature, and qualified referrals for the treatment of eating disorders.

National Association of Anorexia Nervosa & Associated Disorders,
P.O. Box 7
Highland Park, IL 60035
(847) 831-3438

American Anorexia Nervosa/Bulimia Association
293 Central Park West, Suite #1R
New York, NY 10024
(212) 501-8351

National Eating Disorder Organization
Laureate Eating Disorder Unit
6655 South Yale Avenue
Tulsa, OK 74136
(918) 481-4044

Some of the comprehensive treatment centers available include:

Eating Disorders Clinic
The New York State Psychiatric Institute
Columbia-Presbyterian Medical Center
722 West 168th Street
New York, NY 10032
(212) 960-5746

*Treatment is free for individuals who meet criteria for this research program.

Eating Disorder Program
The Cornell Medical Center-Westchester Division
21 Bloomingdale Road
White Plains, NY 10605
(914) 997-5875

The Renfrew Center
475 Spring Lane
Philadelphia, PA 19128
(800) 736-3739
(215) 482-5353

The Least You Need to Know

➤ Anorexia nervosa is a life threatening eating disorder that involves self-induced starvation and refusal to maintain a normal healthy weight for height.

➤ Bulimia nervosa is a serious eating disorder that involves repeated episodes of rapidly consuming large quantities of food, and then ridding the body of the excess calories by self-induced vomiting, laxatives or diuretic abuse, or prolonged exercising.

➤ Compulsive overeating is repeatedly eating excessive amounts of food. Unlike bulimics, compulsive overeaters do not purge and therefore tend to be extremely overweight.

➤ Treating an eating disorder generally requires a collaborative team approach from a psychiatrist or psychologist, a physician, and a nutritionist.

More Fun and Nutritious Recipes

Jam in Popovers

Serves eight

1 cup flour	$1/4$ teaspoon salt
1 cup 1% low-fat milk	1 tablespoon canola oil
1 egg	non-stick vegetable spray
1 teaspoon baking powder	jam or preserves

Preheat oven to 425°. Use non-stick vegetable spray on muffin tin (or popover tin). Measure out all ingredients and pour into a blender. Blend well. Next, pour mixture into prepared muffin tray, filling each tin only $1/2$ to $2/3$ of the way. Bake 25–35 minutes until sides are rigid and top is puffed.

Each popover with an additional teaspoon of jam (optional), is the equivalent of one serving. Serve with plenty of fresh fruit.

Nutrient Analysis for One Serving

Calories 112, Total Fat 3 grams

Saturated Fat .5 grams, Fiber 0.5 grams

Protein 3 grams, Sodium 136 mg, Cholesterol 28 mg

*From the kitchen of Meg Fein

Breakfast Berry Crepes

Serves four

2 cups whole-grain flour

1 egg, beaten

2 $\frac{1}{2}$ cups low-fat milk

non-stick vegetable spray

$\frac{1}{2}$ cup blueberries

$\frac{1}{2}$ cup raspberries

$\frac{1}{2}$ cup sliced strawberries

Place flour in a bowl and add egg plus 2 cups of milk (save $\frac{1}{2}$ cup). Beat with a wire whisk until all lumps are gone and the mixture is completely smooth. Gradually add the remaining $\frac{1}{2}$ cup of milk to make a thin batter. Use non-stick cooking spray on hot skillet (medium-high temp), and pour enough batter in the pan just to make a large circle. Sprinkle desired amount of fruit on top and press down into the crepe. Cook for approx. 2–3 more minutes and then flip the crepe and cook the other side. Carefully lift onto a plate and roll it up.

Nutrient Analysis for One Serving

Calories 325, Total Fat 4 grams

Saturated Fat 1.6 grams, Fiber 5 grams

Protein 15 grams, Sodium 95 mg, Cholesterol 59 mg

*From the kitchen of Lisa Alexander and Jesse Bauer

Vegetable Soup and PB and J

Serves one

Canned low-sodium vegetable soup, 1 cup

2 slices whole-wheat bread

1 tablespoon peanut butter

1 tablespoon jelly

Open the can of soup and heat. While it's warming up, smear the peanut butter on one slice of bread and the jelly on the other. Put them together and what do you get? PB and J with piping hot vegetable soup! An example that healthy eating does not need to be extravagant.

Nutrient Analysis for One Serving

Calories 365, Total Fat 10 grams

Saturated Fat 2 grams, Fiber 10 grams

Protein 11 grams, Sodium 435 mg, Cholesterol 0 mg

*From the kitchen of Pam Shapiro and Dan Schloss

Garden Tostada

Serves four

8 corn tortillas

$^1/_4$ cup nonfat mozzarella

$^1/_4$ cup nonfat sour cream

Salad

$^1/_2$ red bell pepper, chop medium	$^1/_4$ cup chopped scallions
1 anaheim chile pepper, seed and chop medium	4 tablespoons prepared salsa
2 ripe tomatoes, chop medium	2 tablespoons vinegar
2 cups black beans, drained	3 cups shredded dark green lettuce

Preheat oven to 375°. Place corn tortillas on cookie trays—do not overlap. Bake for 5 minutes and turn over. Bake for 10 more minutes or until curled and golden brown. Combine salad ingredients in large mixing bowl. To serve: Place 2 corn tortillas on each plate. Place salad mixture on top of each tortilla. Place 1 tablespoon of nonfat mozzarella and 1 tablespoon of sour cream over each tortilla.

Nutrient Analysis for One Serving

Calories 300, Total Fat 2 grams

Saturated Fat 0 grams, Fiber 9 grams

Protein 15 grams, Sodium 200 mg, Cholesterol 0 mg

Copyright by *Food for Health Newsletter*, 1996. Reprinted with their permission.

Curried Chicken and Rice

Serves four

1 1/2 cups water

1 cup chicken broth

1 cup canned crushed tomatoes

1/4 cup dark, seedless raisins

1 teaspoon curry powder

1/2 teaspoon cumin

1 1/4 cups uncooked basmati rice

12 oz. chicken breasts, boneless, skinless, cut into 1/2-inch cubes

2 cups broccoli florets

4 tablespoons nonfat plain yogurt

In a large sauce pan, combine all ingredients *except for chicken, broccoli, and nonfat yogurt.* Bring to a boil, reduce to a simmer (turn stove to medium or medium low), and cook covered for 8 minutes or until liquid is almost evaporated. Add chicken breast and broccoli florets and cook an additional 5 minutes or until chicken is done and rice is tender. It may be necessary to add more water. Serve with nonfat yogurt spooned over the top of each portion.

Nutrient Analysis for One Serving

Calories 370, Total Fat 1 grams

Saturated Fat 0 grams, Fiber 4 grams

Protein 28 grams, Sodium 230 mg, Cholesterol 50 mg

Copyright by *Food for Health Newsletter*, 1996. Reprinted with their permission.

Eggplant Parmigiana

Serves four

1 large eggplant

2 cups corn flake crumbs

pinch cayenne pepper

$^1/_4$ teaspoon garlic powder

1 cup nonfat plain yogurt

olive oil cooking spray

1 cup grated nonfat mozzarella cheese

16 oz. pasta sauce

Preheat oven to 350°. Slice eggplant lengthwise into $^1/_4$-inch thick slices. (It is optimal to get 6 or 8 slices—that way you have 1 $^1/_2$ to 2 slices per person.) Combine corn flake crumbs, cayenne pepper, and garlic powder together in large mixing bowl. Coat eggplant slices with yogurt on both sides then press both sides well into corn flake crumb mixture.

Set coated eggplant on cookie tray sprayed with olive oil cooking spray and spray top of eggplant lightly with olive oil spray. Bake for 15 minutes or until crisp and golden brown. Top with grated nonfat mozzarella and bake an additional 3–5 minutes until cheese melts. Serve each portion over $^1/_4$ cup hot pasta sauce.

Nutrient Analysis for One Serving

Calories 160, Total Fat 0 grams

Saturated Fat 0 grams, Fiber 4 grams

Protein 11 grams, Sodium 500 mg, Cholesterol 5 mg

Copyright by *Food for Health Newsletter*, 1996. Reprinted with their permission.

Chicken Teriyaki over Linguine

Serves four

Pasta

8 oz. dried linguine noodles

Sauce

vegetable oil cooking spray

12 oz. chicken breast strips (skinless)

1 tablespoons low-sodium soy sauce

2 tablespoons orange juice

1 $1/4$ cups water

3 cups fresh mixed stir-fry vegetables

1 cup snow peas

$1/2$ cup sliced green onion (scallions)

1 tablespoon cornstarch

Cook linguine in 2 quarts rapidly boiling water. Follow package directions for cooking times. Pasta is done when tender but slightly firm in center. Drain in colander.

Make the sauce: Heat a large 12-inch nonstick skillet and spray with vegetable oil cooking spray. Cook chicken strips just until done, approximately 5–7 minutes, set chicken aside. In the same skillet, add the soy sauce, orange juice, and 1 cup water. Bring to a simmer. Add all the vegetables and cook until tender, approximately 6 minutes. Dilute the cornstarch in $1/4$ cup water and stir into the vegetable mixture. Broth should form a light glaze. Add chicken and serve over pasta.

Nutrient Analysis for One Serving

Calories 220, Total Fat 1 grams

Saturated Fat 0 grams, Fiber 9 grams

Protein 25 grams, Sodium 260 mg, Cholesterol 50 mg

Copyright by *Food for Health Newsletter*, 1996. Reprinted with their permission.

Asparagus with Dijon Sauce

Serves four

³/₄ pound fresh asparagus spears

¹/₄ cup reduced-sodium chicken broth

2 teaspoons Dijon mustard or tarragon Dijon mustard

1 tablespoon grated Romano or Asiago cheese

Break woody ends off asparagus and place in skillet. Pour broth over asparagus then cover and steam over medium heat until crisp-tender (about 4 minutes). Remove asparagus to warm serving plate with slotted spatula and keep warm. Add mustard to skillet; increase heat to high and bring to a boil, stirring constantly. Pour over asparagus and sprinkle with cheese.

Microwave Method

Break woody ends off asparagus and place in 2-quart rectangular microwave-safe dish. Pour broth over asparagus; cover with vented plastic wrap and cook on high power 3 to 4 minutes or until crisp-tender. Pour off liquid into 1-cup glass measure. Keep asparagus covered. Whisk mustard into juices. Cook uncovered at high power until boiling, about 30 seconds. Pour over asparagus; sprinkle with cheese.

Nutrient Analysis for One Serving

Calories 20, Total Fat 0.7 grams

Saturated Fat 0.4 grams, Cholesterol 1 mg

©1995, The American Dietetic Association. *"Skim the Fat: A Practical & Up-To-Date Food Guide."* Used by permission.

Traditional Tapioca

Serves four

2 tablespoons quick-cooking tapioca

3 tablespoons sugar

$1/8$ teaspoon salt

1 egg, beaten

2 cups skim milk

$1/2$ teaspoon vanilla

Mix all ingredients (except vanilla) in a saucepan. Let stand 5 minutes. Bring to a full boil, stirring constantly. Remove from heat. Stir in vanilla. Stir again after 20 minutes. Chill.

Nutrient Analysis for One Serving

Calories 115, Total Fat 1.5 grams

Saturated Fat 0.5 grams, Cholesterol 55 mg

©1995, The American Dietetic Association. *"Skim the Fat: A Practical & Up-To-Date Food Guide."* Used by permission.

Cinnamon Apple Phyllo Rolls

1 box of phyllo dough, room temperature
(you'll only need 3 strips)

3–4 medium sized apples (cleaned, peeled, seeded, coarsely chopped, and rinsed in water and lemon juice)

1 tablespoons margarine

$^1/_4$ cup sugar

$^1/_4$ cup brown sugar

$^1/_2$ teaspoon cinnamon

$^1/_4$ teaspoon cloves (optional)

$^1/_2$ teaspoon vanilla

non-stick vegetable spray

Melt margarine in a skillet and add apples, sugar, spices, and vanilla, stirring often. Cook until tender. Remove from heat and let it cool to room temperature. Preheat oven to 400°. Take 3 sheets of phyllo dough and cut them into $^1/_2$- or $^1/_3$-sheet strips. Lightly spray over each group of strips with non-stick vegetable spray, spoon apple mixture onto the strips, and roll up. Place them on a cookie sheet seam-side down, and again lightly gloss the outer phyllo with non-stick cooking spray. Bake 20–30 minutes, until lightly browned.

Nutrient Analysis for One Serving

Calories 274, Total Fat 4 grams

Saturated Fat .5 grams, Fiber 2 grams

Protein 2 grams, Sodium 175 mg, Cholesterol 0 mg

*From the kitchen of Meg Fein

Caribbean Rice Salad

Serves four

Rice

1 $^1/_2$ cups white long grain rice

2 $^1/_4$ cups water

Dressing

2 tablespoons cider vinegar

2 tablespoons orange juice

4 tablespoons nonfat italian salad dressing

Salad

1 15 $^1/_4$ oz. can black beans, drained and rinsed

1 orange, peel, remove seeds, and dice into $^1/_2$-inch cubes

1 mango, peel, remove pit, and chop into $^1/_2$-inch cubes

1 fresh tomato, dice into $^1/_2$-inch cubes

$^1/_2$ jalapeno pepper, remove seeds and veins, mince fine

$^1/_2$ red bell pepper, remove seeds and slice into thin strips

$^1/_4$ cup sliced green onions

6 cups shredded dark green lettuce

Prepare long grain rice according to package directions. If you are in a hurry, use instant rice instead. Allow to cool to room temperature. (This process can be hurried by putting the cooked rice in your freezer in a shallow pan.)

Combine dressing ingredients together and toss with salad ingredients; toss with rice and serve. Additional orange segments and pepper strips may be used for garnish but are optional. Divide entire tossed salad between 4 plates and serve.

Nutrient Analysis for One Serving

Calories 340, Total Fat 1 grams

Saturated Fat 0 grams, Fiber 8 grams

Protein 11 grams, Sodium 230 mg, Cholesterol 0 mg

Copyright by *Food for Health Newsletter*, 1996. Reprinted with their permission.

*From the kitchen of Ellen Schloss

Sweet Potato Stew

Serves six

$^1/_2$ tablespoon margarine

2 cups fresh sweet potatoes, cooked and sliced

8-ounce can crushed pineapple in natural juice

$^1/_4$ teaspoon ground cinnamon

$^1/_8$ teaspoon salt

Heat margarine in a large frying pan. Add potato slices and pineapple. Sprinkle with cinnamon and salt. Simmer uncovered until most of the juice has evaporated (about 10 to 15 minutes), turning potato slices several times.

Nutrient Analysis for One Serving ($^1/_2$ cup each)

Calories 135, Total Fat 1.6 grams

Saturated Fat 0.3 grams, Cholesterol 0 mg

©1995, The American Dietetic Association. *"Skim the Fat: A Practical & Up-To-Date Food Guide."* Used by permission.

*From the kitchen of Meredith Gunsberg

Papaya Sorbet

Serves four

1 ripe papaya (1 $\frac{1}{4}$ pounds), diced

$\frac{1}{4}$ cup plain low-fat yogurt

$\frac{1}{2}$ cup light corn syrup

1 teaspoon fresh lime juice

Place papaya in a 9-inch square baking pan and freeze for about 1 hour. Place frozen papaya in food processor with yogurt, corn syrup, and lime juice. Process until smooth. Freeze for at least 1 hour. Makes 2 cups.

Nutrient Analysis for One Serving

Calories 160, Total Fat 0 grams, Cholesterol 1 mg

©1995, The American Dietetic Association. *"Skim the Fat: A Practical & Up-To-Date Food Guide."* Used by permission.

Spicy Poached Pears

Serves four

1 cup apple juice

$^1/_2$ cup cranberry juice cocktail

1 tablespoon orange juice

$^1/_3$ cup water

$^1/_4$ teaspoon ground cloves

$^1/_4$ teaspoon cinnamon

$^1/_8$ teaspoon ground ginger

4 ripe bosc pears, peeled

Pour juice, water, and spices into a deep saucepan; cover and bring to a boil. Trim the bottom off pears, if necessary, so they stand up straight. Remove core. Add pears and simmer uncovered until tender (15–25 minutes, depending on how ripe the pears are). Remove pears and set aside. Cook the remaining liquids over medium-high heat, stirring periodically, until mixture has reduced by half. Drizzle this juice-syrup over pears, and serve while warm, or chill and serve later.

Nutrient Analysis for One Serving

Calories 165, Total Fat 0.7 grams

Saturated Fat 0.1 grams, Cholesterol 0 mg

©1995, The American Dietetic Association. *"Skim the Fat: A Practical & Up-To-Date Food Guide."* Used by permission.

Glossary

ACE   American Council on Exercise.

ACSM   American College of Sports Medicine.

Active lifestyle   Folks who are constantly on the go. They do lots of walking, taking the stairs, playing sports, or regularly working out.

AFAA   Aerobics and Fitness Association of America.

Anaphylactic shock   A life-threatening whole-body allergic reaction to an offending substance. Symptoms include, swelling of the mouth and throat, difficulty breathing, drop in blood pressure, and loss of consciousness. In other words, get help fast!

Anorexia nervosa   A complex psychological disorder characterized by self-induced starvation. Meaning an "appetite loss of nervous origin," people who suffer from this disorder believe they are overweight, despite the fact that they are often skinny to an unhealthy degree.

Antibodies   Large protein molecules that are produced by the body's immune system in response to foreign substances.

Bulimia   Another psychological disorder personified through abnormal eating habits. Meaning "ox-like hunger," people suffering from bulimia are characterized by a viscious cycle of gorging massive amounts of food only to induce vomiting in order to purge the food from their system.

Calorically-dense foods   Foods that provide lots of calories and fat in a relatively small portion size.

Calorie   The amount of energy food provides. The number of calories a food provides is determined by burning it in a device called a calorimeter and measuring the amount of heat produced. One calorie is equal to the amount of energy needed to raise the temperature of one liter of water one degree Celsius. Carbohydrates and protein contain four calories per gram, fat contains nine calories per gram, and alcohol contains seven calories per gram.

Complementary proteins   Two incomplete proteins in a food that compensate for one another's shortfalls when combined.

Complex carbohydrates (complex sugars)   Compounds comprised of long strands of many simple sugars linked together.

Cross conditioner/Cross-country ski machines   A great aerobic exercise that utilizes the entire body and burns tons of calories without any jarring impact. It's also good for quick warm-ups, because it gets the whole body going. There is, however, one catch: learning the movement can be a bit tricky for some people, and let's just say the term "poetry in motion" takes on a whole new meaning.

Diastolic pressure   This number represents the pressure in your arteries while your heart is relaxing between beats. During this relaxation period, your heart is filling up with blood for the next squeeze. Although, both systolic and diastolic numbers are critically important, your doctor may be more concerned with an elevated diastolic number because this indicates that there is increased pressure on the artery walls even when your heart is resting.

Diverticulosis   An illness or condition where tiny pouches (called diverticula) form in the wall of the colon. The condition is often without symptoms, but when the pouches become infected or inflamed, it can be painful. When this happens, the condition is known as diverticulitus, which can cause fever, abdominal pain, and diarrhea.

Empty calories   Calories with no nutritional value.

Essential amino acids   Amino acids that cannot be synthesized by the body. We must get these from outside food sources.

Fat-soluble nutrients   Nutrients that dissolve in fat. Some essential nutrients such as the vitamins A, D, E, and K require fat for circulation and absorption.

Food allergy   An over reaction by the body's immune system, usually triggered by protein-containing foods (i.e., cow's milk, nuts, soybeans, shellfish, eggs, and wheat).

Food intolerance   An adverse reactions to foods that generally do *not* involve the immune system (i.e., lactose intolerance).

Food poisoning   An adverse reaction caused by contaminated food (microorganisms, parasites, or other toxins).

Food sensitivity   A general term used to describe *any* abnormal response to food or food additive.

Free radicals   Unstable, hyper-active atoms that literally trek around your body damaging healthy cells and tissue.

Glucose (also called dextrose)   A simple sugar found in fruits, honey, and vegetables. It is also the substance measured in blood (i.e., blood sugar equals blood glucose).

Hemorrhoid   Painful swelling of a vein in the rectal area.

Homogenized milk   Milk that has been processed to reduce the size of milkfat globules so the cream does not separate and the milk stays consistently smooth and uniform.

Hypertension   The medical term for sustained high blood pressure. Contrary to how this term may sound, it does not refer to being tense, nervous, or hyperactive.

Hyponatremia   Excessive loss of sodium and water due to persistent vomiting, diarrhea, or profuse sweating. In this case both water and salt must be replenished to maintain the correct balance for your body.

Incontinence   The inability to control excretory functions.

Iron toxicity   Although not very common, iron toxicity is a serious problem that occurs from either a genetic abnormality causing the body to store excessive amounts, or the unnecessary over-supplementation of iron. The result can be liver and other organ damage.

Lacto-vegetarians   This group of vegetarians eliminates meat and eggs from their diet but includes all dairy products.

Legume   Vegetables borne in pods of the bean and pea family that are especially rich in complex carbohydrates, protein, and fiber. They supply iron, zinc, magnesium, phosphorous, potassium, and several B-vitamins including folic acid. Because foods that fall into this category provide ample amounts of both complex carbs and protein, they can fit in either the meat and beans group *or* the vegetable group. Legumes you may know by a more common name include black beans, pinto beans, kidney beans, lima beans, navy beans, soybeans (tofu), black-eyed peas, chickpeas (garbonzos), split peas, lentils, nuts, and seeds.

NSCA   National Strength and Conditioning Association.

NASM   National Academy of Sports Medicine.

Ovolacto-vegetarians   This group of vegetarians eliminates all meat from their diet (red meat, poultry, fish and seafood), however, they do include dairy products and eggs.

Pasteurized milk   Milk that has been briefly heated to kill harmful bacteria and then rapidly chilled.

Proteins   Compounds composed of carbon, hydrogen, oxygen, and nitrogen, and arranged as strands of amino acids.

Psuedo vegetarians   This group will not eat meat on the days they decide they're vegetarian, but will, however, inhale hamburgers and steak sandwiches when they get a craving.

Rowing machines   Another good "total-body" workout (and warm-up machine) without any impact. Be sure to get some pointers on technique, there is an easy way to do it and the *right* way to do. Obviously the right way requires a lot more energy, concentration, and muscular effort.

Scurvy   A disease resulting from a deficiency of vitamin C, characterized by bleeding and swollen gums, joint pain, muscle wasting, and bruises. Scurvy is now rare, except among alcoholics, and can be cured by as little as five to seven milligrams of vitamin C.

Sedentary lifestyle   Folks generally have desk jobs, watch lots of TV, and tend to sit around most of the time.

Semi-vegetarians   This group does not eat red meat, but eats most chicken, turkey, and fish, along with all dairy and eggs.

Simple carbohydrates (simple sugars)   Molecules of single sugar units or pairs of small sugar units bonded together.

Stairclimbers   Cardiovascular equipment that provides a very challenging workout with some potential stress to your knees and lower back (listen carefully to your body). This is a more advanced piece of machinery due to the importance of technique, and therefore a base level of stamina and strength is needed to use this machine even on lower levels.

Stationary bikes   Now they come in two flavors: the upright bike (like a regular outdoors bicycle), and the recumbent bike (legs out in front with high bucket seats lending more support for people with lower back pain). Both types of stationary bikes provide effective aerobic workouts that can give your joints a break because they are non-weight bearing activities. Make sure that the tension is not too high and that the seat is not too low. If you are a beginning biker, ask a trainer to help get you into the proper position for an effective workout. When you are ready to pump up the intensity, play around with increasing your speed before increasing the tension.

Systolic pressure   is the top, larger number. This represents the amount of pressure that is in your arteries while your heart contracts (or beats). During this contraction, blood is ejected from the heart and into the blood vessels that travel throughout your body.

Tofu (firm)   This tofu is stiff, dense, and perfect for stir-fry dishes, soups, or anywhere that you want tofu to maintain its shape. A 4-ounce serving of firm tofu supplies 13 grams of protein, 120 milligrams of calcium, and about 40% of your daily iron.

Tofu (silken)   This tofu is creamy and custard-like, and therefore also works well in pureed or blended recipes such as dips, soups, and pies. Silken tofu doesn't provide as much calcium as the more solid tofu varieties (only 40 milligrams), but it is the lowest in fat and is packed with 9 $\frac{1}{2}$ grams of protein per 4-ounce serving.

Tofu (soft)   This tofu provides 9 grams of protein, 130 milligrams of calcium, and a little less than 40% of your daily iron from a 4-ounce serving. Soft tofu is good for dishes that require blended tofu (commonly used in soups).

Treadmills   Cardiovascular equipment that presents light to moderate impact on your joints depending on whether you are running or walking. Walking on a flat grade is a good starting place for beginning exercisers. As fitness and confidence levels build, you can fool around with increasing the incline, and speed.

Vegetarian   A person who substitutes vegetables, nuts, and seeds for meat in a diet. They vary in strictness, from avoiding all animal products to avoiding meat only. Vegetarian groups include: ovolacto, pseudo, semi, and vegan.

Vegans   This is the strictest type of vegetarian (sort of the Pope of all vegetarians). Vegans abstain from eating or using *all* animal products, from eating meat, dairy, and eggs, to wearing wool, silk, or leather. If you're a vegan you'll need to be extra responsible about getting adequate protein, iron, calcium, vitamin D, vitamin B-12, and zinc.

Index

J-K

L

M

S

X-Y-Z

When You're Smart Enough to Know That You Don't Know It All

For all the ups and downs you're sure to encounter in life, The Complete Idiot's Guides give you down-to-earth answers and practical solutions.

Personal Business

The Complete Idiot's Guide to Terrific Business Writing
ISBN: 0-02-861097-0 ▪ $16.95

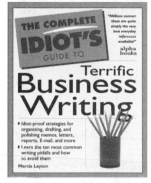

The Complete Idiot's Guide to Winning Through Negotiation
ISBN: 0-02-861037-7 ▪ $16.95

The Complete Idiot's Guide to Managing People
ISBN: 0-02-861036-9 ▪ $18.95

The Complete Idiot's Guide to a Great Retirement
ISBN: 1-56761-601-1 ▪ $16.95

The Complete Idiot's Guide to Protecting Yourself From Everyday Legal Hassles
ISBN: 1-56761-602-X ▪ $16.99

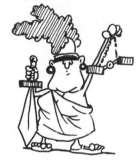

The Complete Idiot's Guide to Surviving Divorce
ISBN: 0-02-861101-2 ▪ $16.95

The Complete Idiot's Guide to Getting the Job You Want
ISBN: 1-56761-608-9 ▪ $24.95

The Complete Idiot's Guide to Managing Your Time
ISBN: 0-02-861039-3 ▪ $14.95

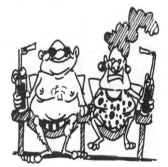

The Complete Idiot's Guide to Speaking in Public with Confidence
ISBN: 0-02-861038-5 ▪ $16.95

The Complete Idiot's Guide to Starting Your Own Business
ISBN: 1-56761-529-5 ▪ $16.99

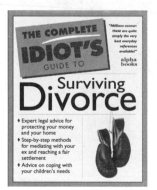

You can handle it!

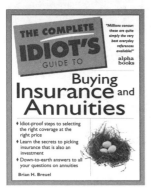
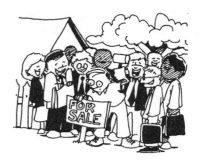
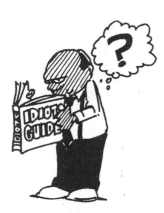
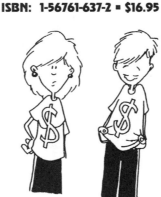
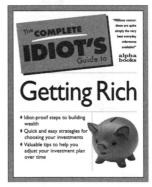

The Complete Idiot's Guide to Learning French on Your Own
ISBN: 0-02-861043-1 ▪ $16.95

The Complete Idiot's Guide to Dating
ISBN: 0-02-861052-0 ▪ $14.95

The Complete Idiot's Guide to Hiking and Camping
ISBN: 0-02-861100-4 ▪ $16.95

The Complete Idiot's Guide to Cooking Basics
ISBN: 1-56761-523-6 ▪ $16.99

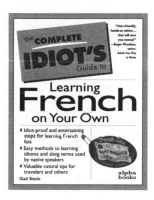

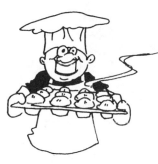

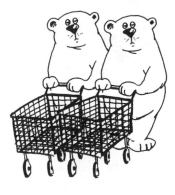

The Complete Idiot's Guide to Learning Spanish on Your Own
ISBN: 0-02-861040-7 ▪ $16.95

The Complete Idiot's Guide to Gambling Like a Pro
ISBN: 0-02-861102-0 ▪ $16.95

The Complete Idiot's Guide to Choosing, Training, and Raising a Dog
ISBN: 0-02-861098-9 ▪ $16.95

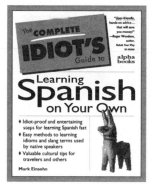

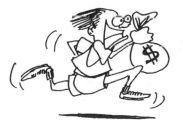

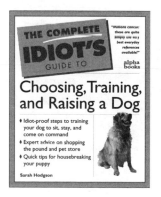

The Complete Idiot's Guide to Trouble-Free Car Care
ISBN: 0-02-861041-5 ▪ $16.95

The Complete Idiot's Guide to the Perfect Wedding
ISBN: 1-56761-532-5 ▪ $16.99

The Complete Idiot's Guide to Getting and Keeping Your Perfect Body
ISBN: 0-286105122 ▪ $16.99

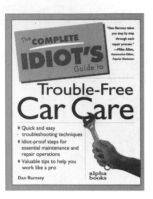

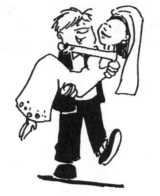

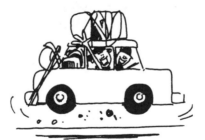

The Complete Idiot's Guide to First Aid Basics
ISBN: 0-02-861099-7 ▪ $16.95

The Complete Idiot's Guide to the Perfect Vacation
ISBN: 1-56761-531-7 ▪ $14.99

The Complete Idiot's Guide to Trouble-Free Home Repair
ISBN: 0-02-861042-3 ▪ $16.95

The Complete Idiot's Guide to Getting into College
ISBN: 1-56761-508-2 ▪ $14.95

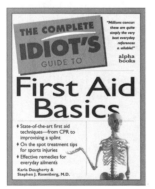

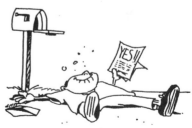